MIGRANTS AND HEALTH

Global Health

Series Editors: Professor Nana K. Poku, John Ferguson Professor, University of Bradford, UK and Dr Robert L. Ostergard, Assistant Professor of Political Science, University of Nevada, Reno

The benefits of globalization are potentially enormous, as a result of the increased sharing of ideas, cultures, life-saving technologies and efficient production processes. Yet globalization is under trial, partly because these benefits are not yet reaching hundreds of millions of the world's poor and partly because globalization has introduced new kinds of international problems and conflicts. Turmoil in one part of the world now spreads rapidly to others, through terrorism, armed conflict, environmental degradation or disease.

This timely series provides a robust and multi-disciplinary assessment of the asymmetrical nature of globalization. Books in the series encompass a variety of areas, including global health and the politics of governance, poverty and insecurity, gender and health and the implications of global pandemics.

Also in the series

The Political Economy of Pharmaceutical Patents
US Sectional Interests and the African Group at the WTO
Sherry S. Marcellin
ISBN 978 1 4094 1214 4

The Politics of AIDS Denialism
South Africa's Failure to Respond
Pieter Fourie and Melissa Meyer
ISBN 978 1 4094 0405 7

Gender and HIV/AIDS
Critical Perspectives from the Developing World
Edited by Jelke Boesten and Nana K. Poku
ISBN 978 0 7546 7269 2

AIDS, South Africa, and the Politics of Knowledge
Jeremy R. Youde
ISBN 978 0 7546 7003 2

AIDS and Governance
Edited by Nana K. Poku, Alan Whiteside and Bjorg Sandkjaer
ISBN 978 0 7546 4579 5

Migrants and Health

Political and Institutional Responses to Cultural Diversity in Health Systems

CHRISTIANE FALGE
Institut für Interkulturelle und Internationale Studien, Germany

CARLO RUZZA
University of Leicester, UK

OLIVER SCHMIDTKE
University of Victoria, Canada

Routledge
Taylor & Francis Group
LONDON AND NEW YORK

First published 2012 by Ashgate Publishing

Published 2016 by Routledge
2 Park Square, Milton Park, Abingdon, Oxon OX14 4RN
711 Third Avenue, New York, NY 10017, USA

Routledge is an imprint of the Taylor & Francis Group, an informa business

British Library Cataloguing in Publication Data
Falge, Christiane.
Migrants and health : political and institutional responses to cultural diversity in health systems. -- (Global health)
1. Transcultural medical care. 2. Immigrants--Medical care--Government policy. 3. Medical policy--Canada--Citizen participation. 4. Medical policy--Germany--Citizen participation. 5. Medical policy--Italy--Citizen participation. 6. Immigrants--Cultural assimilation--Cross-cultural studies.
I. Title II. Series III. Ruzza, Carlo. IV. Schmidtke, Oliver.
362.1'086912-dc23

Library of Congress Cataloging-in-Publication Data
Migrants and health : political and institutional responses to cultural diversity in health systems / edited by Christiane Falge, Carlo Ruzza, and Oliver Schmidtke.
p. cm. -- (Global health)
Includes bibliographical references and index.
ISBN 978-0-7546-7915-8 (hardback)
(ebook) 1. Transcultural medical care. 2. Medical care--Cross-cultural studies. 3. Migrant labor--Medical care. 4. Health services accessibility.
I. Falge, Christiane. II. Ruzza, Carlo. III. Schmidtke, Oliver.
RA418.5.T73M524 2011
362.1086'24--dc23

2011048852

ISBN 9780754679158 (hbk)

Contents

List of Tables		*vii*
Preface		*ix*
List of Abbreviations		*xi*
	Introduction: The Political Fight Over the Accommodation of Cultural Diversity	1
1	Diversity in Health Care—A Discursive Field between Multiculturalism and Universalism	19
2	Community Engagement and Political Advocacy in Canada, Germany, and Italy	41
3	Political Advocacy in the Health Care System	69
4	Barriers in Access to Care *Saime Ozcurumez, Lloy Wylie, Giulia Bigot and Rika Dauth*	105
5	Strategies for Change among Institutional and Civil Society Actors *Saime Ozcurumez and Lloy Wylie*	139
	Conclusion: Political Advocacy and Institutional Change in the Health Care System	177
Bibliography		*185*
Index		*201*

List of Tables

I.1	Migrants' intersection with the policy process	8
I.2	List of interviews conducted in Canada, Germany, and Italy (2006–2008)	15
2.1	Political focus on migrant organizations in Bremen	56
2.2	Degrees of migrants' involvement with policy process compared	64

Preface

This book is based on the work of an international research group whose project *Giving New Subjects a 'Voice': Cultural Diversity in the Health Care System* was funded by the German Volkswagen Foundation (2006–2009). We would like to thank the Volkswagen Foundation for its generous financial support and its laudable commitment to collaborative, multi-disciplinary research. The Volkswagen Foundation`s unique funding scheme allowed for a comprehensive cross-national and conceptually integrated study of the way migrants and their associations interface with the institutional setting of the health care sector and the policy making machinery of different types of states. We are also grateful for its broader funding initiative *Migration and Integration* that provided a most fruitful environment for exchange with other projects and the adjudicators of this initiative.

Comparative research from a trans-Atlantic perspective is truly collaborative in nature. The proposal for the project *Giving New Subjects a 'Voice'* was originally developed by Patrizia Nanz, Carlo Ruzza, and Oliver Schmidtke. National teams under the guidance of Christiane Falge (Germany), Carlo Ruzza (Italy) and Oliver Schmidtke (Canada) conducted the empirical research: Our research groups Christiane Falge (Bremen), Ulla Wittig and Rika Dauth (Leipzig), Giulia Bigot and Maria-Laura Russo (Trento and Naples), and Saime Ozcurumez and Lloy Wylie (Montreal and Vancouver) provided an invaluable service to the project by carrying out research on our cases, conducting interviews, organizing events, and participating in the discussions on interpreting our findings. Christiane Falge was responsible for coordinating the overall research of the three national teams. We also would like to thank our student assistants Sarah Wiebe, Glenn Wigmore, Eleonore Fournier-Tombs, Andrew Bauer, Tom Lindemann, and Cody Willet for supporting us in collecting data, editing texts, and organizing events.

Last but not least, we would like to express our deep gratitude to those representatives from service providers, migrant organizations, and the policy community who were generous with their time and agreed to be interviewed by us. They openly shared their experiences and thus greatly contributed to the success of the project.

List of Abbreviations

ACCÉSSS	Alliance des Communautés Culturelles pour l'Égalite dans la Santé et les Sevices Sociaux
AMIC	Associazione Mediatori Interculturali per la Promozione Sociale
AMSSA	Affiliation of Multicultural Societies and Service Agencies
AN	Alleanza Nazionale
AsylbLG	Asylbewerberleistungsgesetz
AWO	Arbeiter Wohlfahrt
CEPSI	Study Center of International Politics
CGIL	Confederazione Generale Italiana del Lavoro
CIS	Commonwealth of Independent States
CLSC	Centres de santé et de services sociaux
DAB	Dachverband Ausländischer Vereine
DRG	Diagnosis Related Group
FOCSVI	Forum delle Comunità Straniere in Italia
GRIS	Gruppi Regionali Immigrazione e Salute
IBI	Interregional Bank of Interpreters
IFHP	Interim Federal Health Program
IPAP	Institut für Psychosoziale Arbeit und Prävention
ISMU	Iniziative e studi sulla multietnicità
MOSAIC	Multi-Lingual Orientation Service Association for Immigrant Communities
MSSS	Ministry of Health and Social Services
NAC	National Action Committee on the Status of Women
NGO	Non-governmental organization
NHS	National Health System
NPM	New Public Management
ONC	National Coordination Body
PBW	Paritätisches Bildungswerk
PMB	People with a Migration Background
RAA	Regional Office for Questions of Foreigners and Ethnic German Migrants
SIMM	Società Italiana di Medicina delle Migrazioni
SMART	Sharon Martin Community Health Fund
SPT	Straniero Temporaneamente Presente
SSN	Servizio Sanitario Nazionale
STD	Sexually Transmitted Disease
UQAM	Université du Québec à Montréal

VCH	Vancouver Coastal Health Authority
XENOS	EU financed program XENOS integrates activities against discrimination, xenophobia, right-wing radicalism and extremism in Europe.

Introduction: The Political Fight Over the Accommodation of Cultural Diversity

Integrating migrants and minorities into the fabric of society has become one of the critical challenges for contemporary Western societies. Sustained levels of immigration and the irrevocable ethno-cultural pluralization of contemporary Western societies have provoked what is at times a highly controversial debate about the *reasonable accommodation* of newcomers and minorities. Yet, in flagrant contrast to Nathan Glazer's dictum from 1997 that "we are all multiculturalists now," the normative and political underpinnings of multiculturalism have recently been subject to fierce controversy. In particular, in European countries with a strong Republican tradition of Western liberalism, the balance between universal and group-specific citizenship has led to significant struggles over the multicultural aperture of key institutions (such as the educational, labor market and health care systems) and, in some cases, an outright rejection of multiculturalism as a political program. Even in a classical immigrant society like Canada, with its long-standing legacy of multiculturalism, it is far from clear how the state needs to respond to this challenge. Conventional multiculturalist approaches of accepting and integrating migrants have provoked severe criticism and a new debate on what appropriate answers to the underlying structural social and political challenges could be. How does the commitment to welcoming migrants and to publicly recognizing cultural diversity translate into effective and normatively desirable policies? What is the appropriate way of producing and implementing such policies?

What adds to the challenge of *accommodating* migrants and a growing cultural diversity at the beginning of the twenty-first century is that a simple return to assimilationist expectations has also been largely discredited. The outright return to a demand for the uncritical acceptance of the cultural and institutional status quo of the receiving society has been contested and is increasingly difficult to legitimate even in European pluri-ethnic societies. Various initiatives across Europe to facilitate naturalization and combat discrimination reflect this need to address the challenge of cultural diversity more fully.[1] While Dutch authorities seem to have turned their back on multiculturalism as an underlying principle

1 Also conceptually, the simplified framework used to determine which newcomers need to fully integrate into the socio-political fabric of the receiving society is challenged on empirical and normative grounds. See the discussion in Bader 1998; Bauböck 2002a; Benhabib 2002; Cairns et al. 1999; Carens 2000; Entzinger 2003; Favell and Modood 2003; Joppke 2004, 2007; Kymlicka 2001; Parekh 2000.

of regulating integration, the idea of equal inclusion into the universalist French model was seriously challenged as well in the wake of the social unrest in Paris' poorer suburbs in 2005. The situation of disenchanted migrants and in particular their France-born children sheds light on the tenuous promises of the French assimilationist model and a tension-filled reality that is shaped by serious patterns of social and symbolic exclusion. Insufficient incorporation into key institutions such as the educational system, the labor market or the health care system, as well as pertinent patterns of widespread discrimination,[2] have cast a dark shadow on the promises of French-style universalism.[3]

The conundrum of what successful "integration"[4]—or more appropriate the inclusion into different aspects of cultural, social, and political life—has been further highlighted by a profound critique of the legacy of ethnic homogeneity and assimilation in European nation-states. Christian Joppke characterizes the recently introduced "integration tests" and obligatory civic integration courses designed to test the ability and willingness of newcomers to find their place in European societies as a form of imposed assimilation. For Joppke these forms of promoting "integration" are an attempt to engender strong assimilationist pressures on migrants in a top-down manner (Joppke 2007a speaks of a "repressive form of liberalism"). In Europe the theoretically-driven discussion seems to be caught in the polarization between an assimilationist, if not repressive liberalism that perceives of diversity primarily as a genuine threat to its fundamental values and practices on the one hand, and an increasingly manifest awareness of the price that European societies have to pay for not effectively dealing with experiences of exclusion and marginalization of its minorities on the other. Addressing this "crisis of integration," scholarly and public debates alike have deliberated options for conceptualizing integration that successfully tackle the shortcomings of traditional political and policy models: How can we promote a form of social inclusion that recognizes cultural diversity and attending to issues of group-specific social exclusion while at the same time protecting core principles of rights-based individual universalism?

In light of the highly controversial debate on how to effectively accommodate cultural and ethnic diversity it is remarkable to notice the level of abstraction at

2 A recent EU study found widespread evidence of perceived discrimination by migrants in several areas of public life; see EU-Midis (2009).

3 See Kastoryano 2006, and Ossman and Terrio 2006.

4 In discussing the various ways migrants relate to the institutions of the nation-state, we use the term inclusion rather than assimilation or integration. The term inclusion reflects more adequately that highly differentiated societies include individuals with respect to particular functional systems (such as the labor market, welfare, health system, and so on). In contrast, a term such as integration suggests that individuals are included with respect to all facets of their lives into a nationally defined society. In addition, concepts such an integration and assimilation carry a considerable normative baggage and are highly contested in terms of its (social and political) meaning. See for a critical discussion of the concept of integration Pries 2005.

which both the public and the scholarly dialogue take place. There is a surprising lack of empirically grounded, comparative research on what constitutes successful inclusion of minorities, how institutions react to the political claim of recognizing cultural diversity in the public realm, and what stimulates the development of new policies on the ground. We accept the merits of the fundamental equality-versus-diversity debate in evaluating the multiculturalist project, but argue that answers to such questions would be better informed by a more empirically based approach, which can shed light on the practical difficulties and implications of accommodating the plea for the public recognition of cultural diversity. Acknowledging cultural diversity as an important determinant of social and political life is not a good or bad thing in itself; it is not *per se* the source of an irreconcilable clash of civilizations, nor the solution for all problems plaguing the coexistence of different cultural, religious or ethnic orientations. Rather the socio-political effects of multiculturalist policies are shaped by complex institutional responses and learning processes, forms of intercultural dialogue and bargaining processes (Kastoryano 2002). In this respect, we investigate how diversity in a sense of cultural patterns of various migrant groups is written into health care systems; how respective institutional practices deal with the challenge of this type of cultural diversity; how migrants articulate their needs and how these needs gain voice, for example through organizations and advocacy groups.

It is against this background that the main focus of this book has been developed: It presents patterns of changing institutional practices and public policies with a view to the political demands of migrants and minorities to accommodate culturally based claims. We analyze those patterns where the challenges of including cultural diversity in the social fabric are most pronounced: namely, the health care system—a field of political and institutional practice that refers to a central arena of public life. Health care is a critical test case for public institutions' ability to acknowledge and provide room for cultural diversity. It is a sector of public services that migrants are heavily dependent upon. At the same time, it is dominated by rules and practices often alien to those migrants are familiar with from their own countries of origin. In recent years, pro-migrant organizations and anti-racism activists have repeatedly voiced and politicized diversity claims in the health care system. This has given rise to lively political and academic debates about migrants' access to health care and the responsiveness of institutions to their needs.

Furthermore the health care system is a prominent arena for negotiating the status and practical implications of cultural diversity: On the one hand, health care systems adhering to the principle of universal access are often perceived as a beacon of equal rights and entitlements that citizens enjoy regardless of their origin, social status or gender. Equal access to services is a principle that is meant to transcend the internal division of society. This universalist ethics and the promise of equitable delivery of services as a regulatory principle of contemporary health care systems seem to be at odds with the very idea of differentiated access or group-specific special treatment. Yet, on the other hand, there is growing evidence of unequal access to health care services due to class and cultural background of the patients. Migrants and minorities are a particularly vulnerable group. There is ample evidence that migrants are less likely than other citizens to access health-care, especially concerning secondary and tertiary care.[5] The chronic under utilization of services can be interpreted as an issue of failed institutional multicultural opening.

This book then points to a chronic deficiency of several health services to properly address the needs on a relevant and growing sector of the population. As we will show, an already difficult situation is now compounded by new problems related to the aftermath of the 2008 financial crisis and the budget cuts that Western states are imposing on their public services. These are resource problems but they are also cultural problems as the new austerity appears to undermine the political legitimacy of interventions in support of all vulnerable groups and of migrants in particular.

Political Practice as an Integral Part of Migrants' and Minorities' Inclusion

The research whose results this book presents looks at the health sector's responsiveness to the challenge of cultural diversity from a particular, theoretically informed perspective: the authors of this book explore the link between the openness toward institutional reforms in the health care sector to address the issue of cultural diversity openly and effectively and the degree to which migrants and minorities themselves are engaged in deliberating and deciding such reforms. The basic assumption behind this research is that providing those groups with a "voice" in the political and policy process is prone to generate more accepted, effective and appropriate responses to the question how to include newcomers and minorities in the health care sector. In this respect, we suggest to link patterns of political advocacy and mobilization, on the one hand, and processes of socio-political inclusion in key institutional arenas such as health care on the other hand.

Political inclusion is a key component of successfully integrating migrants and minorities into the fabric of a society. The participation of migrants, ethno-cultural groups, and visible minorities in the political process is perceived to be both a yardstick of their degree of inclusion, as well as a way of managing growing diversity within a society. From a theoretical perspective, Tariq Modood (2007) has recently advanced the idea of *civic multiculturalism*, where he calls for a conceptual shift regarding group-related political claims and rights, from an emphasis on cultural identities to one on procedural rules. Under the rubric of civic

5 Adamson et al. 2003; Ali, McDermott and Gravel 2004; Asanin and Wilson 2008; Beiser 2005; Beiser and Stewart 2005; Bowl 2007; Dunn and Dyck 2000; Gagnon 2002; Laroche 2000; McLean et al. 2003; McDonald and Kennedy 2004; Mitra, Jacobsen et al. 2006; Modood et al. 1997; Newbold and Danforth 2003; Schneider et al. 2002; Smith, Matheson et al. 2007; Wittig et al. 2004.

multiculturalism, migrants and minorities would be expected to integrate into a society through exercising various civic, political and social rights but would not be forced into a (culturally) dominant national mode of inclusion. Sites for executing these citizenship rights are not exclusively defined by the state but are also shaped by a multiplicity of actors in civil society, including community organizations, media, and religious communities, all of which act as representatives of migrant and minority groups. These types of civil society actors engage in the public arena, and thus, according to the underlying normative expectations, contribute to the development of mutually beneficial modes of diversity management. From this perspective, civic multiculturalism is "aimed at fostering dialogue, respect for difference, to seeking common ground and negotiated accommodation" (Modood 2007: 130). The hope is that by providing concerned groups with a "voice" in the political and policy process, they will contribute to the development of more legitimate and effective policy responses regarding the political inclusion of newcomers and minorities.

A whole range of—at times conflicting—political aspirations, however, are projected onto the idea of including migrants into the political process. Terms such as civic or community engagement address both the desire of governments for greater efficiency and legitimacy within the policy process, as well as the desire of community groups to act as serious partners in these policy formation processes. The link between integration and political engagement in scholarly debates, however, has predominantly been studied by a perspective "from above," namely with a view to migrants' representation in electoral politics (Bevelander and Pendakur 2009; Gerber 2004; Siemiatycki and Saloojee 2002; Siemiatycki, Rees, Ng and Rahi 2003). Conversely, the issue of community engagement for migrants seems to be harder to grasp and, given the broad spectrum of communal contexts and actors, more difficult to assess in its effects. Another limitation of this past scholarly work is its disproportionate focus on national models of integration and accommodation of diversity (Entzinger and Biezeveld 2003; Favell and Modood 2003; Hollifield 1994; Joppke 1999, 2004, 2007b; Kymlicka 1995, 2001). In this respect, scholarly debate often fails to appreciate that sub-national entities such as regions or cities are also a laboratory for deliberating, developing and implementing multicultural and integration policies (Vasta 2007, Glick Schiller and Caglar 2011).

Accordingly, an urban-centered perspective addresses an under-researched issue in this field includes in its analysis a perspective "from below": the role of governance at different levels of policy-making and the involvement of major community stakeholders in deliberating the political meaning and institutional response to the challenge of accommodating newcomers and minorities. In turn, this perspective raises various research questions: How does the general commitment to the recognition of diversity and the protection of minority group claims turn into initiatives, policies and institutional change in urban contexts, where such issues are most pertinent in day-to-day life? What is the appropriate way of producing and implementing such policies? What kind of "urban citizenship" (Bauböck

2003; Penninx 2009; Rogers and Tillie 2001; Stasiulis and Bakan 2003; Tolley 2003) emerges when migrants and minorities are included in the political process?

Moving away from a state-centered and at times paternalistic approach in which policy initiatives have been conducted also helps to address another endemic problem in accommodating cultural diversity and formulating multicultural rights. From their inception, multicultural policies suffered from a lack of agency of migrants and ethno-cultural minorities.[6] It is the link between including these groups in the decision-making process and giving them a voice in designing social and political change that informs recent discussions on what successful recognition of diversity and integration should look like: Having an equal opportunity to engage in public debate and policy-making is a critical component of successfully integrating migrants into public life, and leads to their inclusion into and acceptance of social institutions and their norms and practices. That is, citizens can recognize themselves in the principles on which such institutions are founded, and develop respect and confidence in them.

Relating this position to practices in the health care system we presuppose that this process of negotiating and validating of institutional practices and its positive effects on including migrants into the socio-political fabric are likely to happen when a space for dialogue and exchange between cultural groups is built into institutional routines.[7] It is this form of political participation of migrants and minorities that promises to effectively address some of the aforementioned contradictions inherent in the current debate on what constitutes a politically feasible and desirable form of multiculturalism. From this perspective, accommodating cultural diversity is not primarily a matter of top-down state regulation but one in which those who are primarily affected are involved in the deliberation on what constitutes multicultural ideas in particular institutional arenas.

With this focus, this book bridges and integrates the relatively isolated fields of scholarly expertise on multiculturalism and cultural diversity on the one hand, and public deliberation, political mobilization and advocacy of migrants on the other. Indeed, equal access to services and opportunities in the public realm for migrants is as much a matter of institutional practices in the health care sector as it is of granting migrants a voice in decision-making processes in broader political terms. Political participation can be seen as an affirmation of citizenship and thus an indicator of successful inclusion. In this latter sense we conceptualize political participation in a dual sense: As a way of assessing migrants' integration and as

6 A good example of this paternalistic legacy of nation states in addressing the thorny issue of integration has recently been discussed by Joppke (2007a). His focus is on civic integration programs that have been introduced in various European countries and that can be interpreted as a hidden attempt to limit allegedly undesirable immigration and to promote state-monitored assimilation.

7 From an anthropological perspective, Frederik Barth (1969) described those as bargaining processes shaping the nature and effects of ethnic boundaries; see on this point also Wimmer (2008).

the very mode in which these processes of integration unfold. In this regard the book focuses on two related aspects: First, it analyzes the channels through which migrants' and minorities' organized interests gain a "voice" in the public debate on accommodating cultural diversity and in the policy-making process. Second, it focuses on processes of institutional change at the level of the health care system and how change is introduced into a realm of public life that, given the legacy of universal health care in the three national case studies (Canada, Germany, and Italy), has been rather hesitant to open up to claims of recognizing group-specific concerns and practices.

Despite frequent restrictions on access to formal politics migrants have become involved in a host of political activities to defend their rights and to press political demands, so that they no longer can be understood merely as objects of political discourse, but also participating subjects (Hargreaves and De Wenden 1993). Regarding the different positions in the political system towards the notion of integration, we have looked at potential causal relations between the intercultural aperture of the national public institutions in the field of the health policy and the level of participation of pro-migrant associations and migrant associations in the policy-making process. To understand how the processes of political advocacy and participation unfold and how they contribute to policy formation with respect to changes in the health care system we are operating with Goffman's concept of frame analysis (Goffman 1974). Based on frame and discourse analysis we investigate the various discursive strategies constructed by health workers, policy-makers and migrant associations about migrants' health access and services. This also includes the analysis of the political discourse concerning the political status of migrants and their appropriate form of socio-political inclusion.[8]

Here it is important to situate political advocacy in a wider context of political claim-making in that they respond to particular, nationally or locally specific political opportunities to gain "voice" in the health care system. The following table provides an overview of the variety of participatory strategies of different actors, and their forms of communication with view to the degree to which they are integrated into the formal policy-making process. Our comparative study allows us to conceptualize political advocacy as an array of organized public efforts ranging from loosely organized, grass-root citizen groups and social movements that have no contact to government or policy-making (defining their protest in sharp opposition to such established institutional actors) to those groups that are—

8 Another theoretical frame that supports our analysis is the literature on political participation, particularly the theory of the structure of political opportunities with the intent to build an interpretative scheme that, at operational level, has proven to be useful to individualize the opportunities of participation for associations. The underlying assumption of this frame is that the degree of structural aperture of political opportunities facilitates and favors the political integration of immigrants (Giugni and Passy 2004; Koopmans et al. 2005).

to various degrees—integrated into networks of health care decision-makers and the policy community.

Table I.1 Migrants' intersection with the policy process

Intersection with policy process	Patterns of participation	Form of communication
No involvement in policy process	Organizing interests of migrant and minority communities; network building in civil society	Raising awareness through exchange of information/dialog at local meetings
↓	Public campaigns	Protest, filing complaints, media campaigns, printed and internet material (framing issues, agenda setting), appearing before public bodies
↓	Participation in health care delivery (organized interests of professionals)	Exchange of best practices; providing advise; drafting recommendations
↓	Informal participation in community outreach/ deliberation	Public exchange with practitioners and policy community
↓	Direct contribution to the establishment of migrant-specific health services (applying for government funding)	Framing of discursive strategies on migrants reduced access to health care
↓	Informal meetings with government representatives	Informal exchange with government representatives
↓	Formal participatory procedure: representation on advisory boards/ councils or policy working groups	Semi-public exchange of information and knowledge with practitioners and decision-maker
High degree of involvement in policy process	Participation in policy deliberation and formal inclusion into policy decision-making process	Deliberation with experts and policy-makers

This schematic summary of the continuum from a loosely organized citizens' initiatives to the formal inclusion into the policy process will serve as a reference point in analyzing the extent and forms of migrant and minority organizations' involvement in thematizing and debating the issue of cultural diversity in the health care sector.

Community Engagement, Civic Inclusion of Migrants, and Policy Change

The idea of promoting community engagement to tackle critical policy issues is neither new nor specific to the concerns of political and social inclusion for migrants (Mowbray 2005). Two trends have been of critical significance with respect to how community engagement relates to issues of civic, social, and political integration of migrants. First, attempts to promote migrants' political engagement resonate with wider trends in contemporary public policy. The involvement of community groups in the policy process is widely perceived to be a key component of the *New Public Management* approach. With its focus on deregulation, accountability, and marketization, this strategy puts considerable emphasis on the role of citizens as clients (Doern and Wilks 1999). While this might not have been its primary target, this approach has contributed to the emergence of more extensive network relationships (Rhodes 2000a, 2000b). The consultation process has been a key element to the success of this market-oriented policy-making that was originally developed in the 1970s in response to concerns about a patronizing state (Marsh 2000). Reflecting this rationale, community engagement contributes to the effectiveness of an approach that is designed to reduce government responsibility, promote a managerial ethos, and stimulate private–public interaction.

A similar logic of policy process restructuring can be detected in the field of settlement services and diversity management. As Hiebert and Sherell (2009) argue in their study of the settlement industry in BC, the task of integrating newcomers to Canada has undergone a process of decentralization in terms of handing down responsibility to the regional and local level (also Edgington et al. 2001). Following a neoliberal logic, this policy field has been transformed by the federal and provincial governments' attempts at outsourcing responsibility for settlement services to community organizations, harnessing the involvement of community groups, and seeking greater efficiency in the spending of public resources. These changes have, however, been coupled with an influx of additional public funding, thereby creating new opportunities to develop multicultural policies and integration programs. The expansion of the settlement sector has gone hand in hand with the decentralization of service provision and the inclusion of local partners in the settlement process. It is with respect to the latter aspect that, to a certain degree, community engagement has played a significant role in the transformation of settlement services across Canada.

Under somewhat different political auspices, and developed as an encompassing device across different policy fields, New Labour in the UK systematically employed community engagement as a vehicle for addressing policy shortcomings and for gaining policy input from marginalized groups (that is, community engagement—combined with substantial budget cuts at the local level—became the central governmental project of the Blair years). At the core of this strategy was a commitment to bringing actors at the sub-national level more fully into the policy process. New Labour's approach to community engagement was driven by the "need to link national policy, regional governance, city strategy and local action in a coherent whole so that top-down and bottom-up initiatives are mutually supportive" (Carley et al. 2000). Beyond a managerial approach to bringing in communities, a normative agenda of good governance, fairer representation of community interests, and civic empowerment provided the—what some critics called rhetorical[9]—rationale for reaching out to community stakeholders (Edwards 2008; Office of the Deputy Prime Minister 2003; Tiesdell and Allmendinger 2001). Based on this comprehensive attempt at policy innovation, key elements of community engagement strategies that have critical relevance to the integration and inclusion of newcomers can be identified:

- *Making policies more appropriate to local, on-the-ground problems*: This orientation is driven by the consideration that effective problem definition and problem solving depends on using local knowledge and expertise. Community engagement is designed to involve local actors by moving beyond traditional barriers between government agencies and community stakeholders. As a result, government policies are expected to gain greater public acceptance and legitimacy.
- *Strengthening the collaboration between different levels of government and community organizations*: A critical aspect of moving policies closer to local communities is the recognition of the importance of sub-national levels of governance, which become decisive in facilitating community inclusion within the policy process. Local governance in particular is entrusted with promoting community partnerships, soliciting input from various civil society actors, and overseeing the implementation of new policies.
- *Strengthening government–citizen relations*: Community engagement involves an important normative claim regarding the democratic character of the governance process. It is conceptualized as a response to growing public mistrust towards government and the need to involve groups who traditionally have been alienated from party politics and government policy-making. In this respect, it resonates with the key findings of social capital literature regarding the growing disconnect between society and public institutions.
- *Active involvement of community representatives*: One key expectation of community engagement is that it is done in a meaningful and open manner. In this respect, engagement ranges from sharing information to active public consultation and participation in the policy decision-making process.

9 Taylor alludes to the criticism that the Blair government faced in this respect: fragmented programs and divisive competition among localities for funds; community involvement that often was more window dressing than a sustained effort to harness the knowledge and energy of local actors; and a systematic marginalizing of elected local councils in regeneration processes, either through top-down directives or reliance on private sector agencies and special purpose bodies (Taylor 2002: 113).

Underlining the conceptual link between community-oriented governance and active participation, King and Cruickshank summarize the key elements of community engagement as follows: for them, appropriate "community development practice" involves

> continuity and sustainability of good engagement, trust and local relationships; opportunities for deliberation; the ability to deal with anger and the legacy of previous poor engagement; tailor-made opportunities for various stakeholder groups to participate; … facilitat[ing] joint influence over issues; mak[ing] use of community 'hubs' and existing communication linkages, understand[ing] the engagement needs and aspirations of community groups and produc[ing] effective engagement networks. (King and Cruickshank 2010: 3)

Their conceptual understanding of community engagement closely reflects the expectations of community organizations to such an initiative. In contrast to perceiving community outreach primarily as a government procedure for a more streamlined and effective policy process, community groups often see it as a genuine opportunity for a meaningful involvement in the decision-making process. From this perspective, community engagement is primarily a vehicle for empowering formerly marginalized groups and for giving a voice to those who are affected by policy decisions. Here the perspective is decisively directed toward grass-roots initiatives and their input into the political and policy process. The underlying idea of community engagement resonates strongly with migrants and minorities who have demanded a stronger say in a process that is programmatically directed at encouraging their inclusion and input yet is often orchestrated in a top-down, state- or elite-dominated manner.

Considering this range of (normative) expectations broad to bear with respect to community engagement, it is worth pointing out that the reach and quality of community engagement is not exclusively shaped by the intentions of the actors involved but also critically by the structural environment in which these processes take place. As we will illustrate with regard to our case studies in a variety of national and local contexts, community engagement processes reflect particular political opportunities, institutional arrangements and the resources that actors have at their disposal. In this respect, the form and results of community engagement are critically dependent on the political–discursive as well material context in which they unfold.

Beyond National Models?

The focus on processes of political engagement is closely related to another conceptual design of the research on which this book reports. We have doubt whether we can paint an adequate picture of migrants' inclusion into the health care system and processes of addressing issues of cultural diversity in the public arena simply by comparing national case studies. In this book we take migrants' access to health care as a yardstick for understanding the multifaceted processes through which they establish social relations and articulate political claims that link them to the various institutions and societal subsystems of the nation-state of settlement (Ager and Strang 2008; Bommes and Geddes 2000; Entzinger and Biezeveld 2003; Haug 2007; Heckmann and Schnapper 2003; Pries 2006). Just like migrants' access to political participation, health care access is both a yardstick of social integration and a measure of attempts by western states to offer an equitable and accessible health system to all members of their heterogeneous population (Sundquist 2001). Our analysis critically examines local variations in access to health care and will situate its results in the ongoing debate about the impact of national versus local settings. For this purpose we also conducted our primary research in a variety of urban centers reflecting a variety of social, cultural, and political contexts at the sub-national level (Vancouver in English-speaking, and Montreal in French-speaking Canada; Bremen in Western and Leipzig in Eastern Germany; Trento in Northern and Naples in Southern Italy).

As a result of globalization and local-level dynamics urban settings vary in several ways despite similar national policies. In this respect we acknowledge cities of different size and different economic setting as significant laboratories for deliberating, developing and implementing multicultural and integration policies. To date, however, the scholarly debate on the challenging issue of accommodating diversity and promoting successful models of integration predominantly revolves around normative debates or competing national models (Bauböck 2002a, 2002b; Entzinger 2003; Parekh 2000). In this perspective local incorporation is only partly determined by national repertoires of citizenship and integration policies while variations between cities of different states are sometimes less significant than between cities within the same state (Glick Schiller and Caglar 2009). As much as national contexts play an important role in developing responses to these challenges, the core idea of this book is to focus on the urban context as an additional and momentous arena for political deliberation and policy formation. This will allow for a better understanding of an as yet under-researched issue in this field: the role of governance at different levels of policy-making and the involvement of main stakeholders in deliberating the political meaning and institutional response to the challenge of accommodating newcomers and minorities in day-to-day practice.

In this regard, this book relates to the broader debate on locality and how it patterns processes of social inclusion. The localized position is framed in a global perspective where migrants' pathways of incorporation are said to vary between cities and their respective positioning within a global economy (Brenner 1999; Caglar and Glick Schiller 2011). City rankings by economists increasingly support this approach by arguing that the economic success of certain European cities is causally linked to their diversity, independent of national policies. Similarly, national integration and citizenship regimes have lost their decisive power to shape patterns of migrant incorporation, and have given way to the local level as the main locus where migrant integration takes shape.[10]

Thus, the working hypothesis is that the sub-national level of governance has developed into meaningful arenas of political debate and policy formation, in which the issues of immigration and integration are addressed more and more frequently. The regions and its cities have also become important laboratories for deliberating, developing and implementing immigration and integration policies (Borkert et al. 2007; Devadason 2007; Hudson 2007; Karapin 1999; Kosic and Triandafyllidou 2005; Vertovec 1998).[11] Considering the new policy competence of these levels of governance in particular in an increasingly integrated European Union, the dynamic of including civil society actors at this level (Jackson 2001), and the relative distance from partisan party politics in the national arena, these regions and cities are said to have become major sites of policy innovation. The approach to these issues varies significantly—so the key assumption—in terms of how these issues are politicized and how processes of public deliberation unfold at these levels of governance.

With this conceptual orientation the book also strives to avoid the traps of methodological nationalism (Glick Schiller and Wimmer 2003) in the following two ways. First, we agree with the shift from a bounded view about society and culture as determined by nation states toward transnationally-oriented research. This shift was basically initiated in the early 1990s, when Glick Schiller and her colleagues brought methodological nationalism into the field of migration research. This critique triggered a perspective on migrants as simultaneously being incorporated to and shaped by receiving and arrival context and since then became increasingly popular (Glick Schiller et al. 2005; Levitt and Glick Schiller

10 With respect to the impact of the nation-state on migrants' pathways of incorporation, the global city literature argued that global cities have decoupled from their nation–states and generalized about migrants modes of incorporation in such cities (Favell and Smith 2006; Sassen 1991; Smith 2001). The majority of migration scholars argue about the determination of migrants' modes of incorporation by national settings. Even if they would acknowledge local variations between cities such as Koopmans (2004), they would argue that cross-national differences are more significant than variations within countries (see also Garbaye 2000). Also gateway city researchers used their local data to discuss migrant incorporation on the nation–state level (see Baumann et al. 2004; Clark 2004; Hiebert 2005; Ley 2004; Waldinger 1996). In their critique against the tradition in migration studies to generalize from the local to the national level, Glick Schiller and Caglar suggest a new approach to urban migration studies by referring to variations in migrant incorporation as a result of a cities scalar positioning (2009). They lament that though several studies have empirically shown the significance of locality (Eade 1997; Mitchell 2003; Ray 2003; Werbner 2002) very few studies have developed a comparative framework about the significance of locality.

11 For the cities in the European context see the EU-funded projects: *Multicultural Democracy and Immigrants Social Capital in Europe: Participation, Organisational Networks* and *Public Policies at the Local Level*; or the *Cities for Local Integration Policies Initiative.*

2004). The global city literature that emerged in this context even argued that cities have become decoupled from their national contexts and have more in common with other global cities than with non-global cities of the same nation-states (Sassen 1991, 2000).[12] It is within this conceptual framework that we highlight considerable local and regional variation within each country in how issues of cultural diversity are tackled and translated into institutional practice.

The territorial reorganization of politics in this field is also mirrored by recent developments in public policy strategies. In this respect our analysis on health care provision turned out as a pertinent example of new public policy strategies and the idea of including citizens more fully in designing and implementing them. The trend toward decentralizing government and strengthening local authority in central public authority areas (Fisher 1998) has created new opportunities for the interaction between groups in civil society and local government with respect to developing and implementing public policies as well as instigating change in the health care's institutional practices (Snavely and Desai 2000; Milewa et al. 2002).

Second, we acknowledge the factual cultural diversity of contemporary Western societies, a diversity that, however, in traditional accounts of multiculturalism is hidden behind images of "homogenous ethno-cultural identities." Identities as markers of group belonging are made subject to a pluralized form of interest formation and deliberation. Such a conceptualization of ethnicity opens new analytical perspectives: It serves not only to move the research approach beyond the orthodoxy of the nation-state and the way it has shaped our basic conceptual understanding of ethnicity and ethnic groups in migration research. If ethnicity is fundamentally conceived as a relational category (Baumann 1996: 19) whose meaning is established in classificatory practices of groups the analytical lens shifts to the contexts in which these boundaries are reproduced and given significance. From this angle, it is no longer the ethnic group with its allegedly given cultural identity that forms the starting point of the inquiry but the way in which groups create and make use of ethnic or cultural boundary markers in particular institutional arenas (see also Barth 1969).

Methodology: In-Depth Interviews and Frame Analysis

In methodological terms our research raised several challenges related to the difficulty of comparing different political systems and studying actors operating in different languages and cultures. To address these issues we have utilized a multi-method approach. This consisted in in-depth interviews with policy-makers at national, regional and local level; civil society personnel working in generalist

12 The global city critique went even further by arguing that globalization affects cities unequally and that a division into global and non-global cities would overlook the different ways specific cities cope with and are affected by globalization (Glick Schiller and Caglar 2009).

associations and in sectoral associations, doctors and other medical personnel and a small sample of users (for the number of interviews with different actors see table below). Secondly, we conducted participant observation and in this context attended meetings of support groups. Thirdly we examined policy documents and content-analyzed them using the methodology of frame analysis. Fourthly several interviews were partially transcribed and we content-analyzed them using the frame analysis approach. Given the relatively small sample of interviews and text analyzed and the qualitative nature of our studies, we refrained from using the limited quantitative data we acquired preferring instead to focus on identifying and discussing prevalent positions expressed by interviewees and recurrent frames. Here a short explanation of the methodology of frame analysis is provided.

Table I.2 List of interviews conducted in Canada, Germany, and Italy (2006–2008)[13]

	Canada		Germany		Italy*	
	Montreal	*Vancouver*	*Bremen*	*Leipzig*	*Trento*	*Naples*
Service providers/ health care sector	6	8	18	8	7	8
Migrant organizations/ NGOs	10	6	12	7	14	12
Policy actors/ Ministries	8	8	11	5	5	4
Experts (professional and academic)	2	3	2	2	3	4

Note: * Some interviews were also conducted in Milan and Rome.

The methodology of frame analysis we utilized is a type of content analysis of policy documents and of interviews and responded to the need to examine systematically the relationship between the policy agenda advocated by associations and the agenda of policy-makers and political actors. Performing this analysis implied a dynamic exploration of strategic framings and re-framings by competing policy actors diagnosing problems and proposing solutions—a process in which not

13 In order to protect the identity of our interviewees throughout the book we will refer to their organizational or professional background only in a generic format. Often associations or service providers are relatively small and providing their names would allow the reader to attribute interviews to individuals.

infrequently a situation emerges of "solutions chasing problems and problems chasing solutions in the absence of a fixed agenda" (Mazey and Richardson 1997). In other words, in approaching the issue of the health of migrants different political cultures define the problem differently—for instance it could be seen as one of health safety in connection to infectious diseases, or one of injustice whereby some groups of citizens are denied basic rights of access to state services, or one of cross-sectoral diffusion of risk as when for instance poor housing conditions or unsafe employment standards are seen to affect the health of migrants. For each of these categories we devised labels to explore the prevalence of different concepts in our different case studies. However, labels are often not stable and vary across different types of actors and the different political color of the political actors interviewed. This dynamic analysis is discussed in the text when we report the uncertainties, discursive changes of time and strategic uses by political and civil society actors of different concepts. In addition there is a more static and long-term characterization which for instance refer to the prevalence of assimilationist or multiculturalist models. Again our frame analysis has been able to document these differences and we have discussed them in the text. This process has also been examined through a comparative exploration of themes present in programmatic documents on health.

In relation to specific types of actors, our analysis focused on identifying aspirations, examining the perception of problems to be addressed by policies and the criticism of actors involved in the policy process and of normative political principles with a guiding impact on policy-making.

The methodology of frame analysis proved particularly useful as it strives to identify and classify recurrent concepts in policy documents and in interviews and to relate them to specific kinds of actors. It also attempts to identify how these concepts change, merge or differentiate over time and across different types of actors. In practice, the analysis was performed with the help of a small team of researchers which helped by providing an external check to the textual interpretations of the authors. The adoption of the technique of frame analysis comes from a central tradition in social movement research and also in policy analysis which has its roots in the work of Goffman (Goffman 1974; Johnston 1995; Snow 2004; Ruzza 2006).

The selection of the frames resulted from our pilot interviews which identified recurring concepts in all the test cases examined. To produce such a list of frames our team of researchers compared a small sample of documents and excerpts of interviews from each of the locations examined. They then focused on examining documents and excerpts from their own county of residence. The examination of documents was then performed. In the initial phase, following the methodology of grounded theory (Glaser and Strauss 1968) the team concentrated on identifying frames as they emerged in the course of the analysis. Subsequently, especially in the initial stages of our research, we discussed uncertain cases, and in doing so reformulated the definitions in a more appropriate (i.e. easily identifiable) way.

Structure of the Book

The first chapter situates the book in the broader scholarly discussion and introduces a theoretically grounded account of the different discursive strategies that frame issues related to inclusion of migrants and minorities in the health care system. Interviews with experts, practitioners and front line workers conducted in the three countries are analyzed with a view to how access to health care is discussed, mainly regarding the tension between a multiculturalist and a universalistic coding of the issue. There are substantial differences among the national contexts: the respective discursive strategies reflect particular nationally specific political cultures and a specific legacy of dealing with the challenges of immigration and accommodating diversity. The claim is made that processes of accommodating cultural diversity are mediated through distinct national "scripts" that shape the understanding of the challenge and expectations *vis-à-vis* the actors involved. Regional differences between cities do show, however, that we cannot simply generalize from the national to the city level as local policies sometimes deviate from national ones.

The second chapter looks at the role of civil society participation in the public debate on cultural diversity and the degree of access migrant organizations have to the decision-making process in particular in the policy community. Patterns of political advocacy and inclusion of civil society groups into the decision-making process are analyzed as they reflect particular nationally- and locally-specific forms of political culture, party politics and institutional arrangements. The analysis of the actors involved, their organizational forms and aggregation criteria enables us to make some instructive observations about the degree to which migrants and minority groups are able to exercise their citizenship rights and articulate their needs in fields of public policy.

We then focus our attention more closely on political advocacy in the health care system as they materialize in our three national case studies (Chapter 3). This chapter offers a general description of main actors (migrants associations, pro-migrant associations, minority–majority issues, public authorities, insurance companies, and so on) that participate in health care policy-making in the three countries, the types of engagement and its formalization, and an exploration of the agenda setting: Who decides what issues are discussed in the formalized participation processes, which type of participation is envisaged and what structures promote its conduct? The chapter also describes the purpose of participation and responsiveness of decision-makers: what is discussed, which kind of requests groups put forward, what attention they receive from public organizations, and the nature of the relationships among associations and between activists and public organizations. Based on interviews and the evaluation of secondary sources, this chapter produces a nuanced picture of the patterns of political mobilization, policy-making and institutional response in the health care sector in comparative perspective. Particular attention is devoted here to institutional practices and the legal framework of the health care sector.

The fourth chapter provides a critical account of the practices of access to health services and discusses the most pressing issues in recognizing and accommodating diversity in the health care system. It addresses the challenges to equitable access to services that migrants and cultural minorities have to face. Problems of access are discussed on the level of legal inclusion as well as informal practices and institutional regulations shaping the day-to-day practice of the health care sector. Here our focus shifts to the local context of our six cities where health care provision is organized and migrants make their claims about necessary reforms. We are interested in the interaction of local political cultures and national regulatory frameworks, the presence of "institutional activists" whose priorities, biases and political cultures color local decision-making processes, and the allocation of resources (see Ellis and Almgren 2009).

The fifth chapter analyzes the strategies adopted by actors to influence change in terms of an "intercultural aperture" of the health care system. Who or what are the main actors involved in promoting change in the health care sector? What are strategies for improving health services for migrants and minorities? Particular examples of triggering political and institutional reforms are analyzed with a view to how issues are approached and how the "voice" of those affected becomes heard. Here the focus is on the action strategies of both migrant or minority advocacy groups and actors within the health care sector (organized interests of nurses, doctors, health care managers, and so on). What strategies have been adopted considering the variety of national and local contexts studied in the context of the research for this book? What strategies have resonated with public sector and policy authorities? How was this change achieved and what kind of new services have been introduced into the health care system? These questions are also addressed with a view to successful examples of how institutional change was achieved and examples of best practices in the health care system. Here the focus will be on varying levels of intercultural aperture in the three countries, best practices of service provision, the quality of care and the challenges that providing service to migrants entails. Using the six urban case studies, authors consider the format, extent and quality of services for these groups, along with issues of equality and patterns of discrimination built into the practices of health delivery.

The concluding chapter will spell out the generalizable findings of the project on two levels: First, it will develop a comparative framework for better understanding processes of political advocacy by migrant groups. Patterns of political mobilization, their interaction with established institutions and policy actors as well as political opportunities specific to the health care sector will be spelled out. Second, it will outline what kind of challenges and success stories the task of including migrants in the health care sector has generated. Both points will be integrated into an interpretative framework that highlights the link between political participation and successful patterns of social inclusion.

Chapter 1
Diversity in Health Care—A Discursive Field between Multiculturalism and Universalism

The Grand Debate on the Effects of Multiculturalism

In research on migration, the debate on how to include newcomers into society and accommodate cultural diversity[1] takes place primarily as a normative debate and on a remarkable level of abstraction. The scholarly community is essentially split between two camps with opposing views about the scope and form in which the state should develop policies to address the challenges of increasingly pluri-ethnic societies. On the one hand, there are those who defend individual-based liberal universalism against any attempt to introduce group-specific entitlements and legal rights. For this group (most prominently Barry 1991, 1995, 2002; Esser 2004; Offe 1998), the multicultural agenda of specifying groups' rights on the basis of cultural identities is fundamentally incompatible with the egalitarian principle of liberalism. Any attempt to challenge liberalism's individually-based notion of universalistic rights and fairness on cultural grounds is perceived to undermine the very notion of a social and political community built on the egalitarian virtues of modern democracy.

In its social and political effects, the "politics of difference," or multiculturalism, is said to open a Pandora's Box of group-specific claims, setting the stage for a dangerous anti-universalism. At the core of this perception is the idea that the specific cultural or ethnic composition of a community[2] is of no (positive) constitutive relevance for individuals. Instead, multiculturalism represents a normatively illegitimate threat to individual autonomy as well as

1 Our comprehensive notion of diversity is based on a multidimensional understanding developed by Parekh, comprising the three aspects of sub-cultural, perspective and communal diversity. Sub-cultural diversity relates to different belief systems and practices in specific areas of life; perspective diversity signifies intellectual ideas about the design of society as a whole; and communal diversity relates primarily to newcomers with their respective belief systems and practices (see Parekh 2000: 4).

2 In our use of the term "immigrant community" as opposed to "receiving society," we are referring to a group of immigrants that collectively identifies through shared belonging, transnational ties, common origin, language and partly shared cultural practices. Neither an immigrant community nor a receiving society is homogenous; they both differ internally in terms of socio-economic status, gender and changing values.

an extremely hazardous risk to society as a whole. Accordingly, this conception sees the public recognition and legal empowerment of group rights as a genuine threat to the welfare state and "its social cohesion" (Cheong et al. 2007: 40; Pero and Solomos 2010; Vasta 2007: 21). Therefore, the socio-political implication of this view is to adhere to an implicit or explicit model of assimilation; an expectation that dominant socio-cultural practices and institutions need to be defended as guarantors of freedom, equality and social cohesion defined in terms of national unity.

The opposing position—most prominently represented by Will Kymlicka (1995, 1998) (see also Habermas 1996; Modood 2007)—argues that it is only by publicly recognizing and protecting minority rights that principles such as equality, freedom and justice can be achieved in a pluri-ethnic society. In a somewhat oversimplified way, one can summarize Kymlicka's crucial theoretical idea as follows: the formal principles of individual freedom and autonomy are critically dependent on a *societal culture* to make them work and it is only by relating in a profound way to their community (defined by sharing a culture, language, a territorial homeland, and so on) that individuals can make meaningful choices and take advantage of opportunities. Essentially, Kymlicka seeks to remind liberals that questions of political and socio-economic equality cannot be decoupled from issues of cultural diversity. With this he suggests a sweeping reconceptualization of liberalism in terms of perceiving minority rights as something that concerns the viability of its fundamental values. In line with this critique of liberalism, Gerd Baumann also questions the universalist claims of a concept based on European philosophy. He casts doubt on the conceptualization most multiculturalist discourses apply to culture, which view society as a patchwork of fixed cultural identities. Instead, Baumann calls for an understanding of culture that more resembles an elastic web of crosscutting and always mutually situational identifications.[3]

The opposition between the positions of individual universalism and multiculturalism[4] has been entrenched in scholarly debates as the choice between two fundamentally opposed and incompatible ways of perceiving and reacting to cultural diversity. Yet already at this level of the discussion, some of the difficulties of this debate become apparent: as much as many of the key concepts in the debate—such as culture, integration, accommodation or acculturation—are meant to describe a social reality, they are at the same time highly political, and thus contested notions. In this respect they become part of the reality that they

3 Baumann questions the boundaries between reified cultures and attempts to turn absolute differences into relative differentiations by giving empirical evidence that people strategically use both discourses: "To be a socially competent Southallian is to know when best to reify and when best to relativize difference" (Baumann 1999: 132).

4 The very term "multiculturalism" is subject to a highly controversial debate on its theoretical and practical meaning (see Kymlicka 2001 and Parekh 2000). In the context of this inquiry, it is used with reference to its dual meaning as a policy committed to the public recognition of cultural diversity and as an endorsement of the value of cultural pluralism.

claim to analyze. Specifically, in their popularized versions in public discourse, these notions frame the problem in a particular way, establishing norms and expectations about the way in which the inclusion of migrants and minorities into society ought to evolve.

Next to the underlying normative scripts that the two main approaches promote, there is a problem that is of greater significance for the research question under investigation here. Both positions that are not by accident prominently articulated by (political) philosophers are surprisingly void of suggestions on how these general ideas should inform day-to-day practice on the ground. On the one hand, the advocates of universalism rely on the naïve assumption that the allegedly superior norms and institutions of Western liberal societies could simply master enough authority and require minorities to adapt them. In this respect, the task of accommodating diversity becomes one of a gradual learning process in which minorities need to learn to live up to the expectations of mainstream society. By equating society with culture, this assumption conceptualizes the nation-state as a homogenous unit that is based on an equality which further assumes that its hegemonic core values are universally accepted (Glick Schiller and Wimmer 2002, 2003). This conception largely denies the internal differentiation of societies in nation-states. On the other hand, the advocates of multiculturalism similarly tend to perceive migrants' or minorities' cultures as fixed and inflexible, ignoring that these communities gradually change in contact with other communities (Vasta 2007: 23). Indeed, academic and public discourse tends to reify and legitimize identity constructions by promoting cultural traits as essential to given social groups. From this perception of multicultural society emerges a normatively and empirically critical question: "Who determines (and how) whether somebody is religious, ethnic, or national enough to deserve equal recognition?" (Baumann 1999: 105).

At times, multiculturalist approaches can be similarly vague in specifying how their normative expectations should materialize in practice. It is not by accident that one of the key proponents of multiculturalism, Will Kymlicka, is rather elusive about how the rights of migrant communities should be accommodated, even though he is articulate about the legitimate claims of so-called national minorities. One key reason behind this omission might indeed be that collective identities are not fixed entities that determine a group's sense of community and its entitlements. Rather, group identities are in flux and continuously negotiated in terms of the meaning that cultural, ethnic or religious differences have. Group identities are constructed, reproduced and contested in social interaction; they are subject to strategic decisions and politically-driven boundary constructions (Eder et al. 2001). It is within this conceptual framework—acknowledging the importance of identities for patterns of inclusion and exclusion while being aware of their constructed nature—that we analyze how practices in the health care system are shaped by such competing understandings of the challenge of accommodating diversity.

We argue that although these membership criteria and the related identities on which they are based are constantly changing, they tend to remain relatively stable long enough that in our specific empirical cases they can be assumed as temporary criteria for multicultural entitlements. We posit that their relative stability is a historical variable that we will document in the different societies that we analyze. In normative terms we would then envisage enough group entitlements to shore up identities and provide needed resources but not at the cost of hindering their transformations by crystallizing the policy arrangements on which recognition and redistribution is based.

Accommodating Diversity in the Health Care Sector-Conceptual Challenges

If one starts relating these general debates to the issue of the accommodation of minorities' and migrants' cultural identities in the health care sector, the recognition of cultural diversity in this societal system seems to be a straightforward task at first sight: it is about the recognition of multicultural society as being composed of identities that are simultaneously collective in terms of language, religion and certain cultural practices, and inter-relational toward, as well as shaped by, other groups or individuals. Viewing society in this way would help us to develop institutional practices and, in the case of health care, improve access and service delivery. Yet social reality often proves to be more complex. Some of those whose interests these reforms regularly target, along with other critical voices, contest what is introduced as a multicultural opening of institutional practices.

First, there is the question of what acknowledging ethnic-cultural diversity in the health care system is meant to look like. On the one hand, old imperatives of assimilation (advancing the simple adoption of so-called "mainstream cultural norms" and the corresponding loss of cultural distinctiveness) have become questionable and no longer provide a valuable path to allow for successful integration of migrants (Alba and Nee 2003). By bringing the concept of methodological nationalism to migration theory, Wimmer and Glick Schiller question the very concept of integration and the way it is based on a container model of state and society (Wimmer and Glick Schiller 2003). The experience of socio-economic, socio-spatial and symbolic exclusion, as well as perceived opportunity deprivation, has generated discontent and disenchantment, particularly among visible minorities. Yet on the other hand, the notion of differentiating access and entitlements for citizens on the grounds of ethnic or cultural identities appears to be in conflict with some basic principles of modern Western societies. The idea of universal, individually-based rights and the status of equal citizens are normative principles that form the basis of contemporary liberal democracies. Empowering cultural groups actually empowers the elites of each culture, privileging their personal visions of what multiculturalism is about. Thus, it might involve perpetuating hierarchies (Barry 2002; Okin 1999) as defined by a culturalist avant-garde, rather than by the common people whom these groups claim to speak for.

Second, the issue of access and proper services in the health care system is only partly shaped by belonging to a particular ethno-cultural or religious group (Laroche 2000). Individuals' socio-economic status or family structures can also be critical factors in this respect. Migrants are often affected by a mix of racial discrimination, material deprivation and patriarchal power structures that have been recognized only to a very small degree by policy-making or even larger public discourse concerning how to tackle the thorny question of providing adequate medical services. As we will further elaborate later in the book, the regularly precarious legal or socio-economic status of migrants is a particularly important determinant of access to adequate services.

The third central problem in implementing such multicultural rights and institutional reforms is a state-centered (and at times paternalistic) approach. From their inception, multicultural policies suffered from a lack of agency for migrants and cultural minorities. Besides the lack of agency, migrants are also described as lacking social capital, explained as a result of a low level of cohesion with the receiving society. However, for lack of empirical data we have little evidence about receiving societies with its cross cutting class and gender boundaries to be more socially cohesive than migrant communities. Besides, assumptions about agency and social cohesion as harmonious community relations are naïve in a context where people are confronted with institutional racism (Cheong 2007: 40) and persistent forms of social exclusion.

By conducting a discourse analysis of the interviews with health experts in our national cases, this chapter analyses how the issue of cultural diversity is framed and conceptualized as an issue that does or does not deserve institutional and political reform. We also show how group identities and cultural differences are discursively imbued with a host of controversial and competing meanings. In particular, we focus on arguments justifying approaches that are based on individual universalism and multiculturalism, and the way these arguments are articulated in the health care systems of countries with respectively specific migration histories and traditions. Here we refer to the theoretical debate on the relationship between individual freedom and a *societal culture* (Kymlicka 1995), relating it to the challenges of accommodating diversity in the health care sector. Essentially, the arguments oscillate between a multiculturalist position which asserts that proper access can only be guaranteed by recognizing the group identity of individuals and the universalist claim that freedom and equality need to be exclusively based on individual rights.

In this chapter we will highlight how, from the perspective of those who work in the system, different understandings and expectations of what constitutes the successful inclusion of migrants into a system like health care informs practice and constitutes the demand for change. This perspective is informed by the idea that the conceptual understanding of the issue, as it is embedded in discursive practices, critically shapes the normative and practical expectations of those working in the field. We adopt a comparative approach as our analytical tool to shed light on the specificity of how such a general understanding of the issue structures options and approaches in the field of medical service provision. In the following analysis of dominant discursive strategies, we seek to detect the dominant understanding of the status of the multicultural challenge in health care by comparing our three national case studies. This study will be organized around an analysis of the competing meanings assigned to the two central concepts of the debate: universalism and multiculturalism.[5]

Constructing the Challenge of Diversity in National Contexts as a Discursive Field

As much as our understanding of—and the political meaning attributed to—cultural diversity is constructed in discursive practices, it is subject to specific national cultural traditions. The meaning of key terms in the debate varies considerably across national contexts. On the most basic level, the meaning of the term "multicultural" or "multiculturalism" is subject to nationally-specific understandings and expectations. For instance, we found that in the European context our interviewees often used this term in a strictly empirical-descriptive sense. It is meant to depict the social reality of cultural diversity in contemporary society without necessarily denoting any normative or political expectation. From this perspective, "multicultural" is simply meant to refer to the *de facto* degree of ethnic and cultural diversity.[6] The discursive arena for discussing such issues is radically different in the Canadian context. Here, "multiculturalism" represents a concept that is inextricably linked to the political project of accommodating diversity as it was launched in the Trudeau era of the late 1960s and early 1970s. Using the term "multicultural" in a conversation thus explicitly or implicitly entails the idea of a state-sponsored program to publicly recognize and protect minorities. In the Canadian context, the term evokes notions of normative and judicial entitlement.[7] The interviews that were conducted in Vancouver and Montreal highlight the degree to which the task of accommodating diversity has come to shape public discourse and establish an expectation in all policy fields

5 The following analysis is based on interviews with political authorities, service providers and representatives of migrant/minority organizations in Canada, Germany and Italy.

6 A good illustration of this is the statement of a hospital directing head-nurse: Her claim "We have always been multicultural" relates to the mere physical presence of immigrants in the German health care system.

7 In 1982, the Canadian Charter of Rights and Freedoms was introduced with the cardinal aim of modernizing the relationship between individuals and the state. At its core, the Charter is a bill of rights that, as one of its major achievements, explicitly recognizes a sequence of group rights worth protecting (Abu-Laban and Nieguth 2000). Among those are rights for linguistic minorities, cultural minorities and Aboriginal peoples that are meant to complement the list of rights and freedoms assigned to individuals in the first sections of the Charter.

(including health care) that cannot simply be negated by service providers or the policy community on the ground.

In order to understand the following analysis of discourses on multiculturalism and universalism, it is worth considering the seemingly obvious: Germany and Italy do not have a similar history of entrenching the rights of minorities in policy practices and, equally importantly, they do not share a distinct multicultural ethos portraying cultural diversity as a positive, enriching component of contemporary society. Against this backdrop it is not surprising to find that the very term "multicultural" is subject to far wider sets of meaning and, in terms of its practical meaning, political projections. The very principle of dealing with diversity in societies that, such as in Italy, have been countries of emigration until very recently is conceptually and politically highly contested.[8] Similarly in Germany, with the exception of the experiment of the Office of Multiculturalism in Frankfurt, there is no established political, legal or social practice providing a commonly shared sense of what multiculturalism represents or what exactly it demands from those involved in the policy process of providing services in the health care sector.[9]

Against this backdrop it does not come as a surprise to note that in both Italy and Germany the debate on multiculturalism is strongly tied to other, more prevalent discourses about key issues that figure large in the Canadian context. For example, a representative of a Vancouver-based immigrant organization summarizes her approach as follows: "Because part of integration is being able to work and be part of a safe and inclusive community, this is where the multiculturalism, anti-racism, human rights aspect comes in" (Migrant Organization, Vancouver, 2006). The mandate of multiculturalism strongly resonates with "universalistic" values of anti-racism and humanism (the link between the two will be subject to a more detailed discussion towards the end of the chapter). In terms of the "meta-narrative"[10] in our European cases, this basic perception of "multiculturalism" is shaped far more strongly by fears of undermining universally applicable rights and entitlements through the introduction of "special privileges" for specific cultural groups. Throughout the interviews from Naples and Trento in particular, there is a recurrent reference to the alleged threat of "ghettoization" or illegitimate "ethnic privileges." At the most abstract level of framing the issue, our interviews from Germany and Italy showed there is the strong assumption that introducing multicultural principles would inescapably compromise key values

8 It is not by accident that in Italy, for instance, "multicultural" policies—like those in Canada in the 1970s—currently consist of support for the culinary or musical traditions of particular minorities. Since then, Canada has moved to define multiculturalism far more robustly in terms of concrete social and political entitlements for its minorities (see Foster 1998).

9 There were, however, several declarations by health experts engaged in claim-making for migrant-friendly health care structures, such as the "*Sonnenberger Leitlinien*" for migrant-friendly mental health care and the "*Stuttgarter Impulse zur kulturellen Vielfalt*" as a guideline for general migrant-friendly health care.

10 See Snow and Benford 1992.

of their political culture, namely equality and fundamental rights. This normative orientation informs the description of the issue of diversity in the health sector in the Italian context. Reference is constantly made to the risk of "ethnicizing access" to the system, which is depicted as being in fundamental disagreement with the health care system and its claims to be based on universal access. One interviewee, a medical doctor from Trento, summarizes this concern in a representative fashion. She suggests that:

> (I) in order to create a multicultural service one would have to develop a type of service that provides responses to each type of culture, which is quite complex and I would not even know if it would be helpful. 'Intercultural' means instead to take into account the diversity of cultures when structuring a health service and how such a service could cross various cultures; how responses to health needs can be formulated when crossing cultures. A multicultural approach would not be useful—(we need instead) a health system that takes into account different medical traditions and the different medical practices of different cultures. By 'intercultural' I mean ways to find answers within our health service which would be suitable to people from different cultures. Answers that take into account the diversity of cultures when addressing their requests, which is different from creating health services according to the culture of origin. (Medical doctor, Trento, 2007)

The reference to "interculturalism" is critical, as it denotes a shift in what accommodating difference in the health care system is supposed to mean in its practical implications. While, in the account of the interviewee, multicultural responses would create culture or group specific services, an intercultural approach is designed to respect diversity without compromising the values of the Italian health system.[11] The overall goal is described to "integrate" migrants into the system and not to create separate services based on belonging to certain groups. A medical doctor from Naples puts this belief in the ultimate superiority of the universal health care system that is allegedly threatened by a multicultural agenda in even stronger terms. For him, differentiating services based on group belonging is prone to produce a "segregated," if not "ghettoized" system.

> In general I am opposed to a mode of ghettoized way of living; I think that we need to learn to live together. Surely, always with a view to the differences that are present; the homogenization is not a good thing; differentiation may be yes,

11 In this respect, the approach is comparable to the one that is currently favored in Quebec, where, according to the recent influential Taylor-Bouchart Commission, an intercultural approach holds more promise for finding a compromise between concerns about cultural marginalization of Canada's French-speaking population and the claims of minorities in and newcomers to Quebec society.

> but not segregation. We should be differentiated according to what is sensible but not as a fact that only applies to foreigners. (Medical doctor, Naples, 2007)

Understanding the general openness to address issues of cultural diversity, while at the same time insisting on the integrity of the universalistic system (which newcomers are expected to accept), has to be also seen against the backdrop of the health care system as a project of the leftist-leaning welfare state tradition of the country. Universal access to the health care system is a historic achievement that is perceived to be under threat by the multiculturalist agenda of making this system more responsive to cultural diversity. Most of civil society's advocates of migrants' rights in Italy belong to the leftist, universalistic tradition and most of the support groups with ties to the Catholic Church operate in the basis of a similar pretext of universal inclusion and individual entitlement (Pero 2005). In our two national contexts from Europe, it becomes evident that positions skeptical of a multicultural recognition of diversity are not only rooted in right-wing, anti-immigrant sentiments, but also in a leftist or religious discourse on universal rights.

A comparable discourse shapes the perception of these issues in the German context. The case of Bremen demonstrates strong reservations about the political participation of the multicultural agenda, which is particularly shaped by the strong leftist, social-democratic tradition in this city state. Interestingly, this universalistic tradition is prone to promote, at least indirectly, a request for assimilation.[12] Particularly for the Social Democrats, who have governed Bremen for decades, differentiating social and political rights along cultural lines is perceived as antithetical to its plea for egalitarian inclusion. Some multiculturalist discourses also draw boundaries by referring to mutual respect of religious and cultural boundaries. One example is the migrant-friendly Catholic hospital, which claims symbolic representation rights, such as the right for crosses to appear on hospital walls. Here, the multicultural agenda gets very close to the universalist claim to grant individual rights. Though multiculturalist in its orientation, this discursive frame is also wary of essentializing migrants' competence. This concern is expressed by a front line hospital worker, who has a first generation background of migration: "It is a big mistake to believe that migrants with a professional background can do a better job" (hospital social worker, Bremen, 2008).

Another prominent concern that could be detected in the interviews from Germany is the assumption that by culturalizing differences, multiculturalism ignores individual difference. The universalist discourse deconstructs multiculturalism based on the assumption that barriers occur in relation to language and poverty; beyond these two structural determinants that are not specific to

12 Joppke (2007 a and b) has recently framed this as the assimilationist underpinning of liberal democracies, which tend to operate with unspoken expectations that migrants have to meet. In this respect he speaks of a "repressive form of liberalism."

migrants or minorities this discourse considers access to be equally available.[13] It also argues that multiculturalism tends to exaggerate differences. A social worker from a mental hospital views staff with a migrant origin as potential assets in terms of cultural sensitivity. However, this asset should not lead to mistaken assumptions about the inherent sensitivity of migrants *sui generis*. Based on their experience with migrant patients, hospital staff arguing in this frame emphasize that individual differences may transcend collective differences. An example could be differing levels of emancipation among female patients with a migrant background, some being more independent while others communicate through their husbands.

Based on a monocultural and monolingual approach to society, this discourse perceives assimilation as a condition for successful access. "Integration" is not viewed as a mutual process; rather, it is a migrant's obligation. What we have encountered recurrently in our interviews from Germany and Italy is the tendency to individualize the issue. From this perspective, access essentially becomes a problem that can only be solved by individuals' cultural dispositions and educational and social resources.

Most universalist quotes consider language acquisition as the number one asset for the successful inclusion into—and the only facilitator for access to—the health care system. This discursive frame subscribes the responsibility for lowering access barriers solely to migrants, who are obligated to acquire the host country's language. For instance: "Not to learn the German language is a serious deficit of migrants who in this way withdraw themselves from the possibility to integrate" (hospital social worker, Bremen, 2006). As part of this discourse, people insist on politicians' responsibility to put more pressure on migrants' efforts for language acquisition prior to and upon arrival in the receiving country. Besides, the discourse is characterized by a claim for assimilation: "I expect from them that they adapt! One has to do that if one goes to another culture" (Hospital head nurse). Arguing for the dissolution of cultural difference, this assimilationist claim denies the need for diversity training and migrant-friendly structures: "I am not responsible for the language problems of people who live here since 20 years and barely speak the language; then it is hard to understand when people get frustrated about me. I have to defend myself against that" (hospital head nurse, Bremen, 2006).

In its attempt to accommodate diversity, Germany is generally presented as too generous to migrants as compared to other "less generous countries." This discourse is not entirely alien in Canada. It is framed in terms of assigning responsibility for failed integration to migrants and minorities:

13 We are summarizing the dominant discourses that emerged from our interviews with health experts. It should be noted that this discourse is not representative of the German health care experts and that nevertheless Germany has experienced streams of claim-making for migrant-friendly health care structures. These streams however do not represent the majority discourse.

> The difference is not in the access the immigrants have, but in their attitudes. Asians are go-getters and want to learn about the system and learn French. They have an easier time accessing health care than, for example, North Africans, who expect everything to be handed to them on a silver platter and don't make an effort to find out what they need to know. (Service provider, Montreal, 2006)

The issue is here framed in terms of welfare state dependence and the related attitude of passivity on the part of those who receive state services. This discourse is embedded in a neo-liberal critique of state intervention which seeks to shift responsibility from society and the state to individual migrants. Still, while articulated by one interviewee, this attitude is marginal in the Canadian sample.

In contrast to the Canadian case, where state-sponsored multicultural policies have created expectations and entitlements in terms of institutional reform, in Germany and Italy such changes targeted at including immigrant communities more fully are recurrently under the suspicion of promoting illegitimate forms of differentiation and privilege. In the Canadian case, however, accommodating diversity has widely been accepted as an agenda that is needed to extend the privileges of universal rights and services to immigrant communities and minorities more fully. Addressing their concerns and adapting service delivery accordingly is, at least at the discursive level, a strong normative expectation. The anxiety about undermining principles of equality—a critical feature of the discourse in our two European countries—is hardly present in the Canadian interviews. In Germany and, most articulately, in Italy the issue of universalism in the health care system is clearly framed through the lens of the left–right divide and the issue of universal access, regardless of socio-economic status. Issues of social exclusion that migrants have to endure are debated far more strongly in terms of access to basic citizenship rights rather than to culturally-specific services. Here, the overall frame of reference is the universalism of the egalitarian left and the Catholic Church that focuses on overcoming legal and socio-economic forms of exclusion (Bigot and Fella 2008).

Justification of Intercultural Aperture in the Health Care Sector

In light of the very different discursive contexts in which the issue of cultural diversity in the health care system is discussed in our national case studies, there is a surprising degree of similarity in how some of the key issues are addressed at the level of service provision and day-to-day operation of the health care system. This section will analyze the ways in which challenges on the ground are discursively framed, and how, on the basis of the principal normative and conceptual orientations, they inform practice and expectations for reform in the health care sector.

Equal Access

The dominant way of justifying some degree of introducing multiculturalism—understood as the recognition and protection of cultural diversity—into the health care sector is access to services in all three national case studies. The demand for equal and full access to health care is the frame that can bridge the plea for recognizing diversity with the logic of universal inclusion. Equal access has been the key challenge of modern health systems (traditionally perceived as predominantly a matter of socio-economic inequality) and describing the accommodation of cultural diversity along the same lines provides an opportunity for making it compatible to the system's rationale and *modus operandum*. As the following citation from an interview with a health care worker from Trento underlines, "providing the best possible service" is one of the key standards of success and self-commitment for the health care community. While diversifying services according to group identity is said to undermine integration in the long run, openness for the concerns of migrants and minorities is described as functionally imperative:

> The concept of fairness is close to my heart, both in relation to health and more broadly as an issue of access in principle. So I do not pose the problem of doing things differently, in a more beautiful way, for their own sake, no, we have to offer to our personnel and to those who use our services the best possible service. So, if we need to offer translation services, or if we need to offer mediation services, it is clear that we must provide them. But I would be weary of creating 'Indian reservations'. I think these might solve immediate problems but in the long run they undermine integration. (Health representative, Trento, 2008)

This statement summarizes the attitude of our interviewees in Trento and Naples well. The key idea to tackle the issue is to introduce a "bridge" that would allow migrants to take full and equitable advantage of the benefits that their health care system has to offer. At the end of the above citation, it becomes clear that this project is ultimately meant to promote the successful "integration" of newcomers. "Successful access" is the concept that is employed to square the circle of assimilatory expectations and the limited openness to including selected services for minorities into the health care system.

A similar normative expectation can be detected in the German case. One critical aspect related to the task of offering appropriate services is to question of the parochialism characterizing the system in the country. One of the recurrent frames is the doubt about the legitimacy of traditional ideas of assimilation:

> One cannot claim that one should assimilate completely to the society one lives in and I think that the recognition of different cultures is an important issue. It is about global values. It is not enough to argue with one's own values. We need to develop a global perspective. (Bureau of Public Health, Bremen, 2004)

More pronounced, however, is the discourse claiming the need for intercultural aperture by addressing migrants' structural discrimination and related negative effects on their health status: "There are aggravating circumstances, as immigrants are excluded as outsiders by racism. This can increase the relapse rate" (hospital social worker). This element is closely related to providing appropriate services. If the health conditions and the medical needs of migrants are related to their status as newcomers in society, the medical system is requested to address these health-related issues. What we find in the interviews are two aspects of this claim. The first one addresses the link between the experience of being a migrant or refugee and health issues (which is a prominent feature in discussing issues of mental health). The second aspect relates the socio-economic status of migrants and what kind of obstacles to using health care services might result from societal marginalization (material resources and knowledge). Again, the logic of universal inclusion informing welfare and health care systems is congruent to the claims of accommodating cultural diversity in the day-to-day business of caring for patients.

Multiculturalism is often justified by health experts with a migrant background. This group claims their role as that of cultural brokers who mediate between a host society and newcomers: "I have lived here for 34 years … and I have accommodated many cultural norms, … which I pass to my patients" (hospital psychotherapist, Bremen, 2005). Some members of this group justify multiculturalism via a modernist discourse which asserts that access to state institutions prevents diversion to alternative (harmful) structures such as religious healers: "The higher the barriers, the more people use the structures familiar to them. Most of them want to be treated by the Hodja[14]—not by us" (hospital psychotherapist, Bremen, 2005).

Only a few quotes were oriented toward mutual accommodation in the sense that the inserted group adapts to existing conditions amid changes in the structure of the receiving society. As articulated by a nurse: "Both sides need to learn how to reach consensus in order for it to be bearable to both sides. We need to learn from the others that not everything we do is right" (nurse, Bremen, 2007). While the general trend is toward assimilation, the discourse oscillates between this and a frame in which diversity is tolerated as long as it does not endanger social cohesion and peace: "We are a 'Coherent Society' and the state should try to support that. They can maintain their identity … but we need to see that living together in peace is possible, that our aim is that different migrants groups live here together peacefully" (employee of ministry, Bremen, 2008).

Regardless of the commitment to being sensitive about the claims of cultural minorities, both in Germany and Italy there is an almost univocal reservation against any kind of group-based affirmative action and any vision of what is

14 Hodja refers to a "traditional, religious" healer consulted by many Islamic communities. Hodja's are often consulted in the case of mental illness and their practices are highly criticized by many practitioners in the health care system, considering them as a threat to modern health care.

described in derogatory terms as "ethnic" health care institutions. The logic of justifying more robust institutional reform is more pronounced in Canada, yet the discursive strategy of justifying such reforms is rather similar:

> We think in terms of, okay, you have a population that is needy, that requires services, and for us the important thing is that they're treated equally with the same respect and dignity. So that is what pushes us forward. It's like: 'treat us with dignity and respect.' And it doesn't matter whether the person is African or poor, or whatever. You have to look at them as an individual who requires, who has a need. That's where we're coming from. (Service provider, Vancouver, 2006)

As described in the introductory section, the issue of accommodating diversity in the Canadian context is explicitly framed as being compatible with, if not a necessary complement to universal individual rights. It is in this perspective that the issue of equal access (understood also as a reflection of the particular needs of individual groups) has figured prominently in justifying the recognition and accommodation of cultural diversity in the health care system.

Appropriateness of Care

There is another specificity of the discourse in Vancouver and Montreal that builds on the above-mentioned attempt to frame the issue of cultural diversity in the tradition of individual rights. At the level of providing services, a request of intercultural aperture is described as necessary in terms of offering adequate services:

> There's this idea, we're going to not distinguish on the basis of language, of religion, and everyone is treated equally, and we're going to treat people according to the number of hours of care they need, and this unit is for this number of hours, and this unit is for that number of hours. But I think we have to go beyond that. We have to transcend that. And it's not necessarily a negative discrimination if people of a common culture are allowed to communicate with each other, and maintain those cultural ties, especially when we're dealing with long-term care, we're dealing with the end of life, we're not talking about social integration here, you know, we're beyond that. It's the care we're talking about. (Service provider, Vancouver, 2007)

What we find in this quotation from a service provider is a recurrent discursive practice in our interviews: the ultimate yardstick for evaluating the accommodation of cultural diversity in the health care system is the appropriateness of the care delivered. This can work both ways. First, there is the commitment to providing forms of treatment in a way that becomes accessible to those from a different cultural background. If the health care system is not able to communicate and deliver services to its clients irrespective of where they come from and which group they belong to, it is said to have missed its primary objective. Second, at the same time, the system is expected to avoid forms of "negative discrimination." This refers to the possibility of delivering services to particular cultural groups without maintaining the general standards of the mainstream system. The task of accommodating cultural diversity is here described in terms of a strong egalitarian spirit. Providing equal treatment for all patients is depicted as "transcending" differences between groups.

It is with respect to this point that the Canadian interviews follow a similar discursive logic as, yet at the same time departs from most interviews conducted in Germany and Italy.[15] As is evident in the following quotation from a Multiculturalism Program Coordinator in Vancouver, the regulatory normative principle is "equitable outcomes" for all. This framing resonates strongly with the universalistic and egalitarian spirit that defined the mindset of many of our interviewees in the European context. Yet simultaneously, "addressing cultural issues" is referred to as a key component of the goal of achieving fair and equitable outcomes. When analyzing the interviews conducted in Vancouver and Montreal, this component was one of the recurrent features that we encountered in our search for a pragmatic approach to dealing with culture. Along these lines, accommodating diversity is depicted as a tool or vehicle for addressing the obstacles that migrants and members of particular communities face in accessing health care and receiving adequate services. The justification of multiculturalism is almost exclusively described in these terms, rather than framed in terms of essentialized cultural identities:

> So, so again it's that whole thing about equitable outcomes. People should be able to receive the same standard of care. They might look different, but the standard is still the same … Like if culture is part of what it takes, if, a, acknowledging and addressing cultural issues is what it takes, to get somebody to have an equitable health outcome, that's why you must do it, so it's not, the value is not to culture *per se*, the value is to the equitable outcome. And the things that you need to take into account. So that's maybe another reason why it's not about immigrant health or , you know, like, because it does ultimately in Canada come down to the concepts of come out of human rights and equity. (Service provider, Vancouver, 2006)

The issue is framed very similarly by a Montreal language coordinator. The reference to the term "intercultural" is a peculiarity of the Quebec context, in which, not unlike the European context, there is a far stronger notion of a dominant (French)

15 Demands for an intercultural aperture of key institutions of public life (such as the health care system) have been articulated over the past forty years in Germany as well. Yet in contrast to the Canadian case, this request has been limited to a small pro-migrant lobby, and only very recently has it penetrated mainstream public and political discourse.

culture. Again, the overall objective of accommodating diversity is depicted with reference to "equal quality" for all and the notion that such a strategy would not be detrimental to members of the majority culture, but to the benefit "of all":

> And we speak of diversity; we speak of intercultural, equity, adaptation. The objective at the other end is that the services be of equal quality for all. And, ultimately, I think that there will be an improvement of the quality for all. And that is what people say, often after the training, and that's what repositions also the whole of the quality of their services, and at that moment it's quality for all, whether you are immigrant or not immigrant. (Service provider, Montreal, 2006)

In overall terms, the framing of the issue seems to be very close to the normative defense of universalism in service provision that we witnessed in the European context. Yet in our Canadian interviews, the idea to reconcile the egalitarian spirit of universal access and service provision with sensitivity for cultural diversity produces more tangible discursive devices for practice. As articulated in the following quotation, one element is the plea for material resources to institutionalize this openness for cultural diversity on the ground. For the purpose of this chapter, what is noteworthy about the subsequent statement is not so much the reference to the concrete measure—namely the cultural competency auditing tool—rather, it is the discursive context in which this issue is introduced. The initiative, which provides appropriate services to clients from cultural minorities, is described as a vehicle for self-empowerment. The multicultural health workers are introduced as advocates that assist this group to articulate their needs and demands for the health care system:

> Well, I think that there is—as part of a chain process, it's important to designate resources, staff resources in developing appropriate frameworks, to ensure that your services are accessible, and so forth. A piece that was done, that I was involved in, done by the Ministry of Children and Families here in B.C. was the creation of a cultural competency auditing tool. And this tool, not only defined what cultural competency was, but actually created a tool to assist people, ...—you know, identify strengths and weaknesses and areas where they could put some resources and time managing.
>
> And it's not meant to mean that we have to have health care silos for each community. But a system that's more reflective of our diversity, will absolutely enhance the accessibility of the system. So it's not about one silver bullet—that's one approach and strategy. There's also the need for interpreters and translators available on call, regardless of where you're accessing health care in B.C. You know, there's the multicultural health workers, the advocates working within the system on behalf of the non-English speaking patients. (Migrant Association, Montreal, 2006)

This account, with its emphasis on moderation and cultural competence, already refers to a last key strategy in justifying and depicting multicultural approaches to the health care system, namely: communication and language.

Communication and Language as Challenges to Adequate Services

One recurrent discursive feature in justifying the intercultural aperture in the health care sector in all national contexts was language and communication. In the German context, for instance, most quotes mentioned language as a criterion constraining migrants' access to health care. Most of the main migrant communities were mentioned in terms of access barriers due to language skills: "We have great difficulties with Polish or Russian patients, because they speak very little German or not at all" (hospital social worker, Bremen, 2007).

In particular, people working in the area of mental health would frequently mention the need for staff with a migrant background and foreign language skills, due to serious communication problems: "We have a colleague who speaks Polish who sometimes helps with translations. When we cannot cope at all, we request the internal translation service—if somebody has time. It is not ideal; all very bumpy!" (hospital social worker, Bremen, 2007).

Some quotes put great emphasis on empathy, as well as a certain sensitivity and receptiveness toward migrants' needs. They allude to the need to be open to accommodating cultural practices in the context of patient care (for instance, hospital staff "giving permission to family members to sleep over, allowing family members to attend the delivery room," and so on). Quotes by health staff with a migrant background framed foreign language skills as an asset for employment, given the growing need in their work environment: "When the director realized about my language skills he said: 40 percent of the women in the delivery room do not speak German. You speak Turkish, Kurdish, Persian? Perfect" (midwife, Bremen, 2004).

The following quote from an interviewee in Naples put similar emphasis on linguistic competence and the need to offer language services in the health care system. Beyond the simple availability of the migrant's language, however, there is a more complex understanding of what successful communication with patients entails. It is described as a practice of communication that is prone to develop a more comprehensive understanding of the patient and his or her cultural environment. It is worth noting how closely the interviewee links the ability to communicate properly across linguistic and cultural barriers on the one hand, and providing services (in this case the pathological diagnosis) on the other.

> Perhaps a separate branch (of health services) no, but someone and something need to be created, such as health centers which would devote a little more attention to the issues of these Christians (sic.—used in the broad sense of humans), that these are patients like everyone else, have diseases, such as every Italian. The difference is that in order for us to be able to interact with

> foreigners we need first to talk to them, so first we need the language. But it is not just the language we need. A different language brings different semantic approaches, which is a complex issue. Our medical diagnosis is closely linked to our ability to understand the other's language in a broad sense, in the sense that how can I understand what he/she is trying to say if I do not communicate the circumstances, beliefs, customs, the unspoken culture of origin of the patient. (Medical doctor, Naples, 2006)

The next statement from a Vancouver interview is very similar. Translation and interpreting services are depicted as crucial elements of offering adequate services to clients. The example of the Dula service[16] underlines how proper means of communication are considered imperative. In this case, the Dula service adopted a deliberate strategy to provide as many services in foreign languages as possible:

> One of the things that we really wanted to do, was to provide translation, language, services, but as you probably know, it's prohibitively expensive to get translators. So, we trained our own Dulas, who—right now we have 14 different language groups, so all of our Dulas are bilingual—I don't think we have a single Dula that doesn't speak at least English or another language. So then we match them—say if their language is Punjabi, then we match them with Punjabi-speaking women, so then they also can translate for us, of course not as an official translator, but certainly as a communicator for the woman. Even if the woman speaks English, sometimes it's more comfortable for her in labor to communicate in Punjabi, so we can get the information from the Dula. (Service provider, Vancouver, 2006)

In the same vein, a representative of a Montreal Migrant association suggests that communication is not limited to linguistic issues. Establishing a successful framework for being sensitive toward cultural differences (sensitizing staff, knowledge of other cultures, proper services, etc.) defines successful intercultural aperture in the health care sector:

> If you want to really see a good hospital adapting its services to a multi-ethnic population, go to the Montreal Children's Hospital because they've done a really wonderful job for many, many years. They're very aware of religious practices, food, dietary requirements of different cultures, cultural treatment, diverse cultural treatment adapted to specific families, so they know, they're probably experts when it comes to child's care, children's care. (Migrant Association, Montreal, 2006)

16 A Dula is someone who assists the midwife in attending to the non-medical needs of women in the last stages of their pregnancy and during labor.

In Germany and Italy, we have not found institutionalized efforts in regular services[17] comparable to the level of intercultural aperture practiced in the Montreal hospital (Falge and Zimmermann 2009). Such efforts largely remained on the level of political claims articulated by pro-migrant groups. Putting emphasis on communication is meant to lend a voice to those cultural groups that do not have equitable access to services. One of the recurrent claims made by service providers and immigrant organizations is that the Vancouver Migrant association focuses on a political framework of empowering migrants and minorities in the process of defining appropriate services for the community:

> And so we're finding that the research, community research is actually shifting. In that it's starting to become a little more community focused; inclusive of community. And I think that is really good because research can affect policy, but policy then has, policy what happens at the community level, has to be linked; and for policy to be good, it almost has to come from the community. Because they can identify what's needed. And so, with the research there just has to be the connection between the two. (Migrant Association, Vancouver, 2006)

Here we find an additional and crucial element related to communication that figured prominently in the interviews conducted in Canada. Communication is not only defined as a mode of properly understanding the needs of other cultural groups in the health care system. It is also about including them more actively in the process of deliberating political and institutional reforms, instead of treating them primarily as passive recipients of services. In terms of the practical and policy-related implications, such a wider understanding of communicative inclusion asks for a mode of community outreach that is often considered alien to institutions such as those which provide health care services. As mentioned above, those who work in the sector and have a migrant background themselves have featured prominently in giving voice to the concerns of migrant and minority communities.

Conclusions

The analysis of how the issue of cultural diversity is framed in the interviews conducted in the three countries under investigation leaves us with a somewhat perplexing, albeit revealing finding. Most notably, there are substantial differences among the national contexts and discursive strategies which reflect particular, nationally-specific political cultures and particular legacies of dealing with the challenges of immigration and accommodating diversity. In the German and

17 Several migrant-specific health care institutions exclusively targeting migrants are on the increase in Germany. This is particularly pertinent in the area of mental health care, rehabilitation and elderly care.

Italian context, there is a strong insistence on universalistic values and a distinct fear of undermining principles of individual rights and equality. Service providers, policy-makers and representatives of civil society organizations articulate reservations about group-specific entitlements and services in the health care system, echoing popular images of "ghettoized" communities or a "balkanized" society. This overall discourse of describing the multicultural agenda of accommodating diversity as essentially incompatible with the logic of universal, individual-based access and services generates considerable reservations about considering institutional reforms in terms of an intercultural aperture. It is based on a very restricted conception of culture, which excludes socio-economic, class, sexual and gender aspects. In the Canadian context, however, this categorical hiatus between multiculturalism and universalism is critically challenged in the discursive practices of stakeholders. In the framing of the issue, the egalitarian spirit of universal service provision and the accommodation of group-specific privileges is hardly a matter of concern. Rather, in the interviews the integrity of the former is portrayed to be essentially dependent on the introduction of the latter.

However, this somewhat over-simplified and generalized demarcation between the "philosophical" discourses on both sides of the Atlantic needs to be taken with some caution on two levels. First, analyzing our material along the overall multiculturalist claim that proper access can only be guaranteed by recognizing the group identity of individuals and the universalist claim that freedom and equality need to be exclusively based on individual rights, we found that the boundaries between the two discourses were partly blurred and oscillating. In several cases the same person shifted between the two categories by partly emphasizing and partly relativizing cultural identities. In this respect, stakeholders in the health care system also reproduce a conceptual ambivalence in the broader political-philosophical debate about what the dividing line and relationship between multiculturalism and universalism is. The ambivalence in what constitutes the basic principles of these concepts and how they are expected to be translated into practice in the health care sector provides a laboratory for inventing strategies for accommodating diversity on the ground.

This leads us to the second element. While the discourse is shaped by the logic of opposing, if not incompatible claims, when they are translated into what they mean in practice, much of this alleged gap between the two ways of conceptualizing the thorny issue of cultural diversity in the health care system disappears. While broader frames in public debate constitute a discursive universe that guide actors understanding of the issue and structure their professional mode of conduct, there are also other factors shaping practices in the health care system. Individual action is likely to be driven also by pragmatic concerns related to the access to, or provision of services in a particular local context. Furthermore, the very process of articulating these concerns publicly and politicizing them is a critical determinant of how these issues are taken up in the daily practice of accommodating diversity in the health care system. In this respect, the discursive environment matters. It contributes to defining the issue, the need for action and possible institutional responses to the challenge. It is against the backdrop of this observation that the following chapter will look at how the task of accommodating cultural diversity unfolds in concrete institutional and political (in our case, urban) settings.

Chapter 2
Community Engagement and Political Advocacy in Canada, Germany, and Italy

Introduction: Accommodating Diversity and Political Participation

The participation of migrants and minorities in public life is a potentially promising path toward incorporating them into different social and political arenas (Castles and Davidson 2000). The literature also widely recognizes the symbolic value of social and political participation as a means of facilitating the process of inclusion in communal life and allowing this group to assert their need for improvement of their living conditions (Fennema and Tillie 1999; Mowbray 2005). However, for several years international research has documented migrants' low participation in the political life of the host country and their modest impact on the decision-making processes that affect them.[1] The implementation of migration and integration policies are commonly conducted with a *top-down* approach that emphasizes the role of public administrations, judicial authorities (Guiraudon 1998; Joppke 1998) and political elites that are able to control decision-making with regard to *immigration policies* (control policies) and further isolate the theme of immigration from public opinion in order to not lose electoral consensus (Freeman 1995, 1998, 2006; Messina 1987, 1989, 2006).

There are, however, significant variations in forms of political participation across countries and modes of participation. This chapter will examine blockages to one aspect of migrants' political participation: their associational participation both in general and in the field of health care and health advocacy. To fully understand these constraints on participation, in addition to examining dynamics directly pertaining to the health sector, one has to look at the general political (discursively and institutionally-shaped) opportunity structure for migrants' advocacy and associational representation in the host societies under investigation. In this chapter, we will first examine the role of political advocacy

1 A fundamental analytical distinction necessary to understanding and describing the political participation of migrants is to differentiate collective actions between "internal" (or infra-political) strategies and "external" (or political-organizational) strategies. Infra-political strategies are "invisible" forms of mobilization because they are aimed at the inside of one's own group in order to gain power and control over it. According to Bousetta's research (2001), these types of strategies are still the most widespread among migrant communities. Political-organizational strategies are instead aimed at the external world and are meant to influence the political agenda (Bousetta 2000).

in general, then turn our focus to the forms migrant advocacy takes in our three national case studies.

Research on patterns of political participation has recently focused on emerging *bottom-up* political activism and pressure in relation to the shaping of immigration policies. Where migrant communities have deeper roots and are present in greater numbers, and where they have voting rights and the legislation is more open to the influence of citizens' groups, changes are notable at both the individual and collective level. Migrants and minorities have become more visible and more organized at the political level, enhancing their capacity to make political claims, particularly in urban contexts (Garbaye 2005; Martiniello 2006; Martiniello and Statham 1999; Schrover and Vermeulen 2005).

Martiniello points out various factors that have an impact on the political integration of migrants (2006: 84). If, in the initial phase of immigration, the level of political integration is influenced by factors such as short-term economic objectives, or reflects a level of political engagement that is very limited in terms of its impact on policy-making (Martiniello 2006), the dynamic of integration is more likely influenced by more complex factors. Therefore, according to Martiniello, it would be inappropriate to interpret migrants' passivity in terms of apolitical attitudes; behind an apparent lack of commitment, active or implicit forms of political engagement could be disguised (Martiniello 2006: 87).

On the one hand, the level of political inclusion could depend on the identification of migrants with the receiving society and at the level of the democratic norms and values adopted by migrants. The level of participation depends on:

> … their ideas and political values, on their previous involvement in politics (including experiences in the country of origin), on the degree of institutional richness of the migrants' ethnic communities, on their views on temporary or permanent presence in the place of residence, on their knowledge of the political system and its institutions, on the social capital and on the density of *networks* of migrants' associations. This is in addition to the typical determinants of political behavior, such as the level of education, the linguistic skills, the socio-economic status, gender and age or cohort factors. (Martiniello 2006: 58)

On the other hand, political integration can depend on c) the rights guaranteed to migrants in the guest society and d) on the political opportunities for participation, mobilization and representation. The ability of migrants to organize collective action (and the forms their organizations take) is strongly influenced not only by their access to citizens' rights and to the electoral process (Koopmans et al. 2005), but also by the political opportunities guaranteed by the host countries (Fennema and Tillie 2001; Ireland 1994). Of critical importance in this respect are the openness and ability of local and national authorities to: adopt measures to address cultural diversity; implement and sustain such initiatives effectively; stimulate institutional representational forms; and facilitate the transformation of migrant groups from informal networks to associations (Bousetta 2000; Statham et al. 2005; Martiniello 1998; Penninx 2004; Soysal 1994).

All these factors, however, also interact with the organizational ability of migrants. Notably, their social capital (Putnam 1995), and in relation to it their ability to form and consolidate associations, provides them with skills to interact with and achieve favorable policy outcomes from the policy framework of the host society. In addition migrants' engagement and political advocacy are critically dependent on a favorable socio-cultural climate. As we will see in the following, the political struggle over proper access to health care is decisively structured by forms of discrimination and a political climate that in particular over the last years has been shaped by strong anti-immigrant rhetoric. This chapter considers these factors and their impact on the main typologies of collective action (migrant associations/ pro-migrant associations/ ethnic communities/ public authorities/ insurance companies/ and so on) that influence health-related policy-making in the three countries. We provide an exploration of agenda setting processes, such as: who decides which issues are discussed in the structured processes of participation; which are the strategies and the institutional practices adopted in the health systems in order to institutionalize the interests of migrants in the *policy-making process* (the types of engagement and its formalization); how the requests for participation in the policy-making process are expressed by associations and the subsequent responsiveness of decision-makers; which kind of requests groups put forward; the purpose of participation; the sense of identification with the *issues* frequently raised among migrants and minorities; the presence and mobilization of groups with a specific social capital; the presence of networks among the subjects interested in the *issue*; and which relationships exist among associations and between activists and public organizations.

The analysis of political participation of migrants and associations that engage in advocating for their interests is limited to a specific type of *immigrant policies*: health policies. The health *policies* field is particularly suited for this type of analysis for several reasons: First, one can identify a substantial gap between acquired rights and their effective fruition within the health system (Conti and Sgritta 2004; Geraci 1996; Morrone and Mazzali 2000). As health care systems are often based on the regulative idea of equal access and universal entitlements, it proves to be challenging to accommodate minorities in terms of their equitable access to services. Second, questions of recognition of migrants' needs are also emerging (although rather slowly) in this field, both in terms of rights of access and fruition, and in terms of special requests advanced by different cultural and ethnic groups. The analysis of actors involved in the field of health care policies, their organizational forms and aggregation criteria enable researchers to make observations on the extent to which immigrant and minority communities are able to exercise their citizenship rights in the three countries under investigation in this book.

To explore the degree to and form in which civil society associations play a role in policy formation and institutional reform in the health care sector, we interpret the impact of civil society actors from a more general perspective as a first step. This will allow us to conceptualize the scope and form of civil society advocacy more systematically, providing the conceptual framework for our analysis of the health sector in chapter three. In this chapter, we focus on structural changes in contemporary politics and policy-making that encourage or provoke the advocacy of civil society actors. In particular, we highlight when participation is framed and conceptualized as an issue that does or does not entail institutional and political change. We identify what kind of understandings and expectations of migrants' participation can be found among the relevant actors, and when participation is seen as potentially able to inform practices and channel claims for policy change. We proceed in two steps: First, we discuss how civil society and policy formation are linked. Second, we relate the involvement of civil society actors to the broader political-cultural environment in which these actors operate in the three national contexts. Focusing on the structural and cultural factors shaping the role of civil society associations, we gain a better contextual understanding for how this plays out in the health care sector.

The Impact of Civil Society on Policy Formulation, Delivery, Implementation and Monitoring

When one speaks of the role of civil society in policy contexts, an array of idealized references, organizations, individuals and roles are often implied—which requires clarification. Sustained social attention to the role and functions of civil society is still relatively new, but some key features of the "civil society" discourse are already changing. Over the last three decades, the impact of civil society formations has been increasing in the policy process of most states and at all territorial levels, and the attempt to include a variety of them in policy consultations and service delivery is ever-expanding in every region of the world (Rosenbaum 2006; Thouez and Channac 2006). Concerns with civil society recur and often refer to two distinctive meanings of the concept: its role as an ideal space of individual-level citizens' activities in the public sphere, and as a set of associations of different kinds. Whilst distinct, these two meanings are at the root of the resurgence of civil society activism and have in common an endeavor to broaden forms of political participation. However, at least in the policy process of most Western states, the idealization of civil society that emerged in the mid-1990s is now being replaced by a more pragmatic experimentation with different models of inclusion of civil society actors. Even at the ideological level, the early, often uncritical glorification of civil society has been substituted by a debate on the advantages and disadvantages of involvement in policy networks and engagement in service delivery activities.

In discussions of civil society, references are often made to an intermediate public space between the state and private individuals and their families, or to the role of associations. In regard to associations, connections are either made with organized private interests (and in this context, with the role of business lobbies and their activities of persuasion and exerting influence on the policy process), or, more frequently, with public interest groups and their role of advocacy or of service delivery (typically the voluntary activities of the third sector). For instance, the latter includes service delivery activities that often replace aspects of the welfare state. References to civil society also include the advocacy activities of public interest groups which attempt to influence the policy process on behalf of particular constituencies, such as gender and ethnic groups, and groups defined by their sexual, political or religious orientation. These groups may also seek to influence the policy process, not on behalf of specific constituencies, but on the basis of universalist values perceived as not sufficiently represented in the electoral arenas.

Although all political actors have endorsed a stronger role for civil society, their reasons and the contexts in which this has come about are quite different. Typically, center-right neoliberal views tend to conceptualize civil society as an instrument to promote freedom of choice and they associate civil society with the market. In contrast, the left sees civil society as an instrument to promote inclusion and redistribution and connects it more closely to advocacy groups and advocacy coalitions (Chambers and Kymlicka 2002). An enhanced role of civil society is extolled by the right because of its anti-state implications (the possibility of exercising political and policy functions outside the state), and by the left because of its potential for redistribution and advocacy activities in favor of marginalized groups (Cohen and Arato 1999).

New Opportunities for Civil Society Organizations in Policy-Making and Public Administration

For the purpose of our research, it is worth spelling out in greater detail the factors that are driving the increased interaction between civil society and the public sector. Among the wide array of functions that the public sector performs, its expenditures on disadvantaged groups vary considerably according to, for instance, the size and regulatory model of the welfare state (Esping-Andersen 1990, 2002); that is, areas in which, among its other tasks, the state implements regulatory activities and allocates resources to disadvantaged groups. Resources for poverty relief, the advancement of gender or racial equality and projects for local development in underprivileged areas are differently central to the policy activities of the state; they are regulated at different levels of governance. Assessing the relations between states and civil society, scholarship has traditionally worked with the notion of distinct (welfare state) models that can be found across Europe. Whilst there are still substantial differences within Europe, there is also a gradual diffusion of public sector models and processes of regulative isomorphism that work over substantial periods of time, creating and diffusing idealized models that civil society incorporates because of needs for legitimacy and pressures for normative compliance (Meyer and Scott 1983). One important general trend in this regard is a gradual process of the state's opening up to external inputs and its growing administrative decentralization. Regulatory interventions and provisions for disadvantaged groups can be implemented within a hierarchical model of state operations that accords with the idealized Weberian model of the Westphalian state (Poggi 1990); yet this is the model that to different extents is ceasing to be the main normative referent. Such interventions and provisions can be delivered through the delegation of services and the acquisition of technical information from market organizations in a competitive framework. States can rely on the substantial involvement of civil society through the donation or purchase of third-sector activism and skills, and regulatory decisions can be taken on the basis of the advocacy of public interest organizations (although it is evident that the involvement of civil society is more important in some policy domains than in others).

One critical example of how civil society organizations have become an increasingly significant part of policy-making is the prominent New Public Management (NPM) approach that, for particular ideological reasons, strongly advocates that NGOs become part of contemporary, market-oriented public administration and governance. Civil society organizations are increasingly part of NPM arrangements (and of a mixed economy of welfare) and are also increasingly assessed on the basis of some of the crucial values of NPM. With its focus on deregulation, accountability, transparency and marketization (Anheier 2009), this strategy puts considerable emphasis on the role of citizens as clients (Doern and Wilks 1999).[2] While this market logic might not have been the primary target of community engagement, this approach has contributed to the emergence of more extensive network relationships (Rhodes 2000 a and b). The consultation process has been a key element to the success of market-oriented policy-making, which was originally developed in the 1970s in response to concerns about a patronizing state (Marsh 2000). Reflecting this rationale, community engagement contributes to the effectiveness of an approach that is designed to reduce government responsibility, promote a managerial ethos and stimulate private–public interaction. In addition, the boundaries between state and non-state actors are weakening: Different mixes of actors are involved in collaborative projects which have sometimes been referred to as "post-bureaucratic" and which indicate a new alliance across the state/non-state divide aimed at shaping social behaviors. This has, for instance, been documented in examples of mixed-actors environmental governance (Gunningham 2009).[3]

2 For the implementation of such public management approaches in the health care sector see Dent 2005; Simonet 2008.

3 Under somewhat different political auspices, and developed as an encompassing device across different policy fields, New Labour in the UK systematically employed community engagement as a vehicle for addressing policy shortcomings and for gaining policy input from marginalized groups (that is community engagement became the central

Interviews with policy-makers in a variety of different administrative contexts suggest that the most important reason for including all civil society groups in policy-making contexts is to acquire information (Walker 1991). Good policies are based on appropriate technical, social and political information. Information is costly and it can become scarce and biased in an under-resourced state. Funds to acquire *information* through scientific research are limited and powerful economic actors can often provide relevant, but not unbiased information. Civil society groups, through their scientists and their grassroots bases, can often provide information that counterbalances the information provided by industrial and business lobbies and can complement the often limited understanding of specific social and territorial contexts that would otherwise be difficult and expensive to study. In a constantly changing political and social environment, public sector activities are aimed at improving the social conditions of a population with frequently changing needs. Empirical research shows that civil society formations are valued primarily for the quality of the information that they can provide. This fact has induced several organizations to develop specific policy, technical, sociological and scientific skills. For instance, at both the local and supranational level, institutionalized environmental groups are often highly specialized and possess specific knowledge on complex sectors such as transportation, agriculture, or energy (Rootes 2007, 2008).

A related factor is that the participation of civil society groups can foster processes of *policy learning* that are useful for the entire public sector. Policy learning can be facilitated by the existence of a thick, associational, inter-organizational field able to produce debating spaces in which deliberative forms of political participation can take place. These spaces do not necessarily need to be consensual and to always result in shared decisions. As interviews with civil servants involved in consultations show (Fishkin 1993), there is a widespread view that conflict is an essential feature of effective decision-making in a democracy. However, it is best expressed and elaborated in a variety of fora—not just the agonistic arena of representative institutions and processes. State actors often argue that their ultimate decision-making power does not diminish the information-providing, preference-aggregating and preference-redefining benefits of involvement in debating fora. Thus, the informational contribution of civil

governmental project of the Blair years). At the core of this strategy was a commitment to bringing actors at the sub-national level more fully into the policy process. New Labour's approach to community engagement was driven by the "need to link national policy, regional governance, city strategy and local action in a coherent whole so that top-down and bottom-up initiatives are mutually supportive" (Carley et al. 2000). Beyond a managerial approach to bringing in communities, a normative agenda of good governance, fairer representation of community interests and civic empowerment provided the (what some critics called rhetorical) rationale for reaching out to community stakeholders (Edwards 2008; Tiesdell and Allmendinger 2001).

society organizations includes a better provision of information on which to base policies and can stimulate better decision-making.

The joint need to acquire information and process it correctly is particularly pressing in some areas, such those previously mentioned: services to migrants; poverty reduction; and local community self-help groups (Rosenbaum 2006: 46). Because it is in these areas that NGOs often concentrate, their contribution is essential. Likewise, *advocacy contribution* and *service delivery skills* in areas related to gender issues are important when the process involves different levels of governance which have institutionalized anti-discriminatory practices selectively. For instance, Rosenbaum points to the case of international donor organizations which use civil society groups for that purpose (Rosenbaum 2006: 47). Similar considerations apply to supranational entities, such as the EU in relation to some member states.

The inclusion of civil society and its contributions to policy-making has to be understood with a view to the distinctive governance architecture. The European Union has a relatively weak center within which member states attempt to affect policy change in a structural situation of European institutions characterized by limited decision-making power, a constantly changing institutional architecture, limited political legitimacy and often poor coordination capacity (Ruzza 2004). In this situation, all interest groups (including public ones) have an important role in supplementing a weak policy process and making up for limited implementation effectiveness. However, it also becomes imperative to overcome the obviously overpowering role of economic interests. For this reason, all European institutions have for many years emphasized and supported the aggregation, professionalization, institutionalization and inclusion of civil society groups.

To summarize, it has been argued that the public sector increasingly needs civil society because it provides benefits that are scarcely available through partial inclusion into the policy-making process. These include: public-sphere communication; information acquisition and diffusion; aggregation of preferences; policy improvement through deliberative policy learning; involvement in governance structures and ability to represent public sector users at various territorial levels; transnational advocacy; and venue-shopping contributions for better policies and resources. Increasingly, public administration is in need of additional resources that only civil society can offer—particularly information, the ability to represent specific social groups and donations of activists' time and energy.

It emerges from the foregoing analysis of the distinguishing traits of civil society organizations that their functions, action repertoires and identities are often closely interlinked. In the public sector, organized civil society performs functions of advocacy, policy-pressure, information-providing, minority-representation, monitoring of policy-making and implementation and political-societal interaction on issues of political communication. In this perspective, classic analyses of the concept of representation in governance structures need to be reconsidered in light of a more articulated interaction between state and non-state political actors and a more articulated role of associations (Pitkin 1967; Warren 2001). Thus, civil society activities can broaden and redefine political space and act on behalf of specific social constituencies. Associations contribute to the welfare of these constituencies by engaging in a variety of interactions with the public sector.

They may choose to engage in these interactions either while seeking autonomy from the state and its territorial articulations, or by seeking involvement. Different civil society formations assess the advantages and disadvantages of institutionalization in different ways. Organizations closer to the un-institutionalized social-movement sector may reject involvement with the public sector, or accept only some forms of involvement. Some organizations have described participation activities as "a tyranny" which, in exchange for resources and influence, engenders compliance and limits the possibility of criticism. Clearly, different types of civil society organizations will exhibit different institutionalization trajectories, different types of inclusion and a different mix of functions in institutional, non-institutional and public sphere settings—the empirical dimensions of this mix of roles would be an important subject for further research. In any event, their task is increasingly facilitated by a very positive emphasis on civil society: A set of consultation practices between policy makers and civil society actors has emerged on a global scale, constituting a new paradigm in policy formation and service delivery at all levels of governance. This transformation has had a critical impact on the health care sector and the role that civil society organizations, specifically those initiated by migrants and pro-migrant groups, play in this arena of public administration and policy-making.

Participation of Migrants in Public Life: Introducing our National Contexts-Changing Perceptions of Migrant Associations

The main dimensions that affect how the political environment supports or penalizes associations are whether they are seen as useful constitutive components of democracy or as unjustified pandering to special interests. This in turn depends on the one hand on how the role of associations is generally conceptualized in different countries, and on the other hand on how migrants are seen as making a necessary contribution or are seen as a hindrance (such as a potential security threat and a source of social strife). As we will argue, our case studies differ substantially on the interaction of these two variables. Having introduced the respective setting of migrants in our case studies, we will review the role of these contextual settings in the political discourse and in the policy practices of our three national case studies.

Migrants' Participation in Canada: The Presence of the State in Promoting Diversity and Multiculturalism

The 1960s and 1970s saw a series of fundamental changes in the way that the Canadian state and society perceived and dealt with immigration and diversity. Three interconnected elements need to be considered for their long-term impact on the political opportunity structure for migrant and minority groups in this country: the presence of the state in promoting diversity and multiculturalism; the active role of civil society and immigrant advocacy groups; and the particular opportunity structure in the local, urban context. These elements will be considered with regard to their impact on promoting and restricting advocacy in the field of cultural diversity and health care.

The momentous decision in the late 1960s to change its immigration policy and to endorse an official policy of multiculturalism led Canada to move away from an orientation toward white Anglo-Saxon immigrants. Newcomers started to be selected based on their qualifications and not on their origin. As a result, Canadian society quickly became the destiny of migrants from around the world, resulting in a high degree of cultural diversity (so-called "visible minorities" are projected to the majority in Canada's metropolitan cities by 2016). The increased diversity of Canadian society was accompanied by the state's public endorsement of cultural, ethnic and religious plurality, as well as a commitment to equal, non-discriminatory treatment of all citizens. A host of policies helped to strengthen the status of newcomers and their legal entitlements.

The first element, next to a rapid process of naturalization (Bloemraad 2002), was a public policy intended to support integration, driven by the idea of turning newcomers into full citizens with equal opportunities as quickly as possible after their arrival in Canada. Integrating migrants into their receiving society was thus defined as an overriding duty of all levels of government, reflecting the mindset of the expanding 1970s welfare state. This task was not simply left to the market or civil society (Abu-Laban and Gabriel 2002). Until this day it has established the sense of legitimate expectations toward the state, which, for instance, is seen as an agency to correct the systematic exclusion of, or discrimination against certain groups.

The second element was the way in which, under the auspices of the multiculturalist creed, the Canadian state came to play a more proactive role in policies of integration and was explicitly committed to promoting cultural diversity as an organizing principle for modern Canadian society (Rummens 2003). Initially, the Trudeau government used state funding for minority groups to protect their cultural heritage and to remove cultural-linguistic barriers to full participation in Canadian life. In the 1980s, this emphasis on supporting these groups in their folkloric activities changed toward addressing wider issues related to racist and discriminatory practices from which minority communities who came to Canada after 1967 were suffering. The 1988 *Multiculturalism Act* officially acknowledged this focus on concerns for equality, identity and justice, and gave it a more solid legal base.

This changed perspective on and commitment to migrants also found recognition in how the Constitution was amended. In 1982, the Canadian Charter of Rights and Freedoms was introduced with the cardinal aim of modernizing the relationship between individuals and the state. At its core, the Charter is a bill of rights that, as one of its major achievements, explicitly recognizes a sequence of group rights worth protecting (Abu-Laban and Nieguth 2000). Among those are rights for linguistic minorities, ethno-cultural minorities and Indigenous peoples which are meant to complement the list of rights and freedoms assigned to individuals in the first sections of the Charter. This gives ethno-cultural minorities in the country a strong legal base from which to demand public recognition of needs attached to their status as a minority. In addition, and perhaps more importantly, this affirmative reference to group rights and the protection of minorities provides these groups with legitimacy and resonance within the country's fundamental normative self-commitment. This proves to be of critical weight in daily political struggles.

If diversity is promoted as Canada's strength and source of innovation, it becomes difficult to justify exempting certain policy areas of public life (such as the health care sector) from demands for the recognition of cultural diversity. In addition, the introduction of bilingual services in Quebec and the commitment to protecting French-speaking communities has set a precedence that cannot be easily neglected when other ethnic groups articulate demands to have their cultural needs recognized and protected in public life and institutions. In this context of multiculturalism, the state is committed to reach out to minorities and to include their political demands (if only at times in a consultative way) in the policy process.

The cities of Vancouver and Montreal are good examples of this structural openness of state agencies to community outreach and consultation (Berthet and Poirier 2000). Quebec's community engagement strategy is centered on the formation of a committee that consults with ethno cultural communities regarding questions concerning health care provision. The committee has been designed as a consultative body and it reports directly to the Minister of Health and Social Services. Its main task is to advise the Minister on the specific health and social service needs of ethno-cultural communities. With its regular meetings at the ministerial level and its broad mandate from community-based groups, the committee is able to publicly voice the concerns of immigrant and minority groups and find some voice in the policy community. However, its role is primarily consultative and its reports and recommendations are not binding to political decision-makers.

There is a notable split between those organizations that are included in the committee and those that refrain from working within the policy process. Being partially included into the policy community (that is being asked to contribute their expertise to debates or to be represented on some policy committees) tends to have a de-radicalizing and socializing effect. It is thus not surprising to note that there is a political rift between those associations that are privileged in terms of their connection to and funding from government authorities, and those that are forced or chose to pursue their goals independently from state agencies.

The Role of Civil Society, Professional Networks and Immigrant-Minority Advocacy Groups

The multicultural project could not have been as successful as it was if it had been orchestrated from a state-centered, top-down approach. The political élite headed by Trudeau's Liberal Party surely initiated it in order to deal more effectively with the cleavages of a pluri-ethnic society, or as some argue, in a mere opportunistic move to capture the votes of French Canadians (Gerber 2004). Yet at the same time, state-centered policies are partly responsible for setting in motion a dynamic that far exceeds the initiatives of the federal government. The experience of recent decades shows how groups in civil society have increasingly engaged in defining the reach and boundaries of group-specific rights. In this respect, multiculturalism has become a kind of political umbrella under which civil rights activists, immigrant and minority advocacy groups, union organizations, parties and business groups have been engaged in determining the meaning of the abstract principles of fostering cultural diversity in actual socio-political terms (Schmidtke 2007). Particularly in the Canadian context, it is striking to see how advocacy groups representing the different migrant communities have become a very articulate and influential voice in the public arena, affecting the political agenda in a way unimaginable in a typical European context. To put this into provocatively candid terms, issues of migration and the related question of identity and equal inclusion have developed into a resourceful political cleavage in contemporary Canadian society. Its underlying normative issues have come to shape much of the country's social movement sector and party politics beyond the activities of migrant or minority lobbying groups.

The federal policy on multiculturalism clearly had an impact on the mobilization of ethno-cultural communities. Particularly in the period after the 1970s and 1980s, federal multiculturalism intended to expand the capacity of migrant communities to take collective responsibility for dealing with the causes of inequality and for developing mobilization strategies, including judicial recourses, in order to be able to exercise their rights at all levels of government (Bradford 2004). The activity of groups in civil society has critically contributed to making diversity and cultural pluralism a principal issue in public debate and, from a normative perspective, a principle greatly endorsed in Canadian society and politics. One example is the social movement sector, where the Canadian women's movement has been strongly affected by issues of diversity. Its anti-discriminatory ethos has made the Canadian women's movement particularly, however by no means exclusively among the social movements, sensitive to issues of racism and minority rights. The National Action Committee on the Status of Women (NAC), as the main organization for women's groups in Canada, adopted an amendment of its constitution in 1991 that required that one of four vice-presidents and other leading positions were reserved for women of color, aboriginal women and women with disabilities. In 1993, Sunera Thobani became the first "visible minority" to be the president of NAC. Her leadership was part of a larger move for the organization, which involved redefining "women's issues" to include issues such as racism, immigration and refugee policy and economic and trade policies. Far from being merely a policy guideline, the idea of a multicultural society is now at the center of public debate and has become a critical reference point in many political battles. In this regard, multiculturalism turned from a celebration of folkloristic differences into a matter of power sharing and deep political cleavages in Canadian society.

In sum, what we can observe in the Canadian case is a somewhat self-reinforcing cycle of ethnic mobilization and political responsiveness of the political system. On a more theoretical level, our assumption is that the active involvement of these groups in the decision-making process, as much as it is often contested and difficult to implement, is a key component of a successful multicultural opening of the health care sector. The ability to voice concern and gain access to decision-making processes is critical to preventing inadequate services and to empowering the structures using them. The gradual cultural opening of the Canadian health care system over the last decade can only be understood in reference to the demands articulated and initiatives launched by civil society groups. It is the recurrent experience of the Canadian example that state programs introducing cultural diversity into the institutional practices of the health care system came about as a result of pressure from within the system itself (professionals), or from immigrant-minority groups denouncing the inadequacy of services for their clientele.

Migrants' Participation in the German Public Life: Hesitation about Political Advocacy of 'Cultural Groups'

On a national level, the support for immigrant organizations is considered an important part of general civil society engagement in Germany. On a regional level, however, the political establishment widely perceives such support to be a genuine threat to democracy. For instance, in 2002 the *Enquete-Kommission* of the Red-Green government underlined prominently that the collective representation of migrants' interests is key to their successful integration into German society: "The public recognition and perception of migrant organizations and projects has not been articulated enough yet insofar as the potential for self-reliance of ethnic communities and their efforts to integration have been underestimated" (Enquete-Kommission 2002).[4] This statement, that the political self-organization of migrants and minorities takes on the role of a bridge between newcomers and the receiving society, is based on a position also prominently held by German scholars working in this field (Bommes 2007; Bommes and Thränhardt 2010; Elwert 1982;

4 Translated by the authors.

Schiffauer et al. 2002; Schönwälder 2010). These political organizations are said to play a "bridging role" in terms of creating familiarity with and trust in institutions of mainstream society. However, a recent study by Schönwälder on migrants' political participation in North Rhine Westphalia has come up with the result that migrants come nowhere close to parity representation in the 29 big cities of the federal state. Schönwälder therefore concludes that although Germany has come to see itself as a country of immigration it is far from achieving the equal political incorporation of all of its citizens (Schönwälder and Kofri 2010; see also Green 2004; Hansen and Koehler 2005; Luedtke 2005; Schmidtke 2004).

Yet at the same time-and this reflects the general political debate about appropriate responses in dealing with cultural diversity in public life—the idea of political mobilization by migrant and minority organizations has sparked some outspokenly negative reaction in public discourse. These organizations have repeatedly been accused of promoting political radicalism. During the 1960s and 1970s, so-called "guest workers" were accused of supporting left-wing extremism; in the 1980s, this concern was more strongly directed against the Grey Wolves (a rightist Turkish nationalist organization). More recently, scholarly and public debate has turned to issues related to Islamic extremism that, in terms of its impact on integration, is described to have fostered a dynamic of exclusion through mainstream German society and the self-exclusion of radical organizations (Ögelman 2003). For instance, one of Germany's most influential scholars in the field of migration studies, Friedrich Heckmann, has talked about the "trap" (Heckmann 1989) into which the political self-organization of migrant groups would lead in terms of a cycle of exclusion and self-exclusion. In a nutshell, this position asserts that independent political organizations for (radical) minorities would actually aggravate the crisis of integration and alienate particular groups even further from mainstream institutions and cultural practices.

Against the backdrop of this debate, it is surprising to realize that there are very few empirically-grounded studies that look into the relationship between migrants' political self-organization and integration. Notable exceptions were the studies that came out of the *Wissenschaftszentrum Berlin*. In their study of Berlin, Berger, Galonska and Koopmans (2004; see also Koopmans and Statham 1999) claim that they have found no evidence that the political participation of migrants poses any threat to political integration in Germany. According to another study, there was no evidence that political participation would lead to uncontrollable "parallel societies" or undesirable forms of political radicalism. On the contrary, they argue that even political participation that is oriented toward the migrant's country of origin is likely to promote political inclusion in Germany, rather than perpetuate forms of exclusion (Koopmans, Berger and Golonska 2002: 28).

However, it is worth noting that Koopman has recently adopted a far more critical perspective on multiculturalism by arguing that multicultural policies tend to erode the welfare state (Koopmans 1999 and Vasta 2007: 20).[5] Here again, the discourse on the alleged effects of migrants on social cohesion is structured by the perception of Islamic values as being opposed to, if not incompatible with "core values" of Western European liberalism. The fact that many migrants are still exposed to social exclusion and marginalization rarely challenges this narrative. Vasta argues that while ethnic identification and religion often become strategies in the fight against racism and marginalization, this is often labeled as "segregation" (Vasta 2007: 19 and 31). Rather than imposing assimilation to avoid these forms of radicalism, however, Parekh's framework of civic multiculturalism puts forward the need for a common sense of belonging. Hence, migrants need to be included more fully into the receiving society and its various institutions through cultural recognition and structural changes that ensure social equality (see also Bauböck 1996: 114; Parekh 2000: 221). The likely outcome of this change in societal structures and institutions is a two-way process based on mutual accommodation (Vasta 2007: 27).

Processes of including migrants and minorities in the political arena have a decisively different trajectory on the city level (in our case, Bremen and Leipzig) and yet show visible differences between cities. Three phases of political participation in civil society can be observed in Bremen. In the 1970s and early 1980s, many migrant organizations that addressed a range of social and political issues were established. Most prominently, they claimed the right to vote (for non-citizen permanent residents) in communal elections, advocated the establishment of a state representative for "foreigners" (*Ausländervertretung*), supported a multi-lingual radio program for migrants and demanded improved access to social services. New forms of political intervention were entertained following the blueprint of the (at the time) popular social movement sector, which included public fora, pamphlets for public debate, informal deliberations with state representatives, and so on. As part of a global salience of religious movements next to an array of new associations, Muslim migrants also started to found mosques. The first was established in 1973, followed by 30 more by the early 1990s. The imams for six of 11 Turkish mosques were recruited in and financed by Turkey. In a similar vein, many Christian migrants started to establish Pentecostal movements and engage themselves in churches.

In contrast to the growing number of mosques and churches, the number of active migrant associations was on the decline during the second phase in the 1990s. These associations gradually lost their presence in the public arena. Since the closure of the Office for Foreigner Affairs (*Amt des Ausländerbeauftragten*) in 1999, the list of migrant organizations in Bremen has not been updated; a reliable estimate of how many are still active is difficult to obtain. During the course of our

5 With view to the disintegrating force of multiculturalism, Koopmans and Statham claim that "indeed the multicultural appetite grows the more you eat; there may ultimately be something to the warnings against a self-sustaining fragmentation of the nation-state that opponents of multiculturalism fear" (1999: 692).

research, we were able to contact over half of the organizations on the 1999 list. Our findings indicate that migrant membership in these organizations had dropped considerably over the course of the 1990s and that many of the old associations had simply ceased to exist.

Almost all of the associations that are still active have a strong orientation toward the country from where the particular migrants emigrated. The majority of the organizations were founded by migrants from Turkey (27 percent), followed by those founded by migrants from the former Soviet Union (17 percent) and sub-Saharan Africa (10 percent). Many of the groups have a strong focus on cultural events such as dance and music (35 percent), and on providing a general and non-issue-specific forum for exchange (28 percent). As is illustrated in the following graph (see Table 2.1), other associations are active in the areas of education, sports, humanitarian aid and gender issues. Considering the Canadian context, it is striking that in Bremen there are hardly any organizations with explicitly political aspirations regarding community and settlement services. This finding can be read as an indication of the degree to which migrants and minorities in Bremen are alienated from the communal organization of these services.

Table 2.1 Political focus on migrant organizations in Bremen

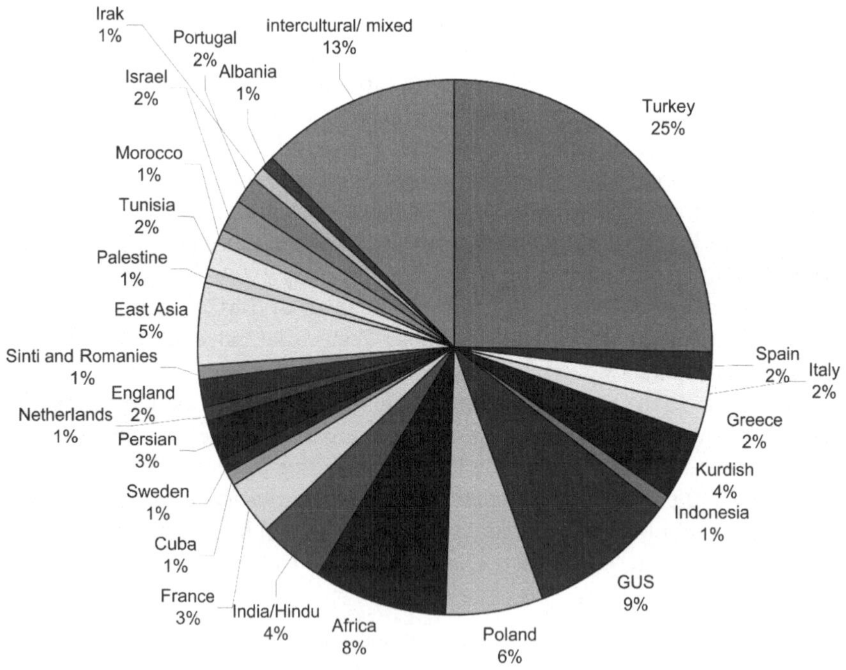

Source: Fieldwork Bremen.

From 1986 to 2004, there was an umbrella organization in Bremen (*Dachverband Ausländischer Vereine, DAB*) that initially was widely supported by an array of collective actors and (state) institutions. Given its close proximity to the Social Democratic Party, however, other parties grew increasingly wary of the DAB. In addition, its focus on the "national orientation" of the Turkish community led to it being increasingly shunned by established national parties. Eventually, corruption allegations and a financial crisis led to the closure of the DAB. The Senate of the city of Bremen interpreted the collapse of this organization as a general failure of the funding scheme for migrant organizations and decided to stop such funding as a result. This in turn put an end to the second phase of migrants' political participation in Bremen.

The third phase was introduced by the recent transformation of Germany's citizenship law: the country's (restricted) attempt to create a modern immigration law and to acknowledge its character as a country of immigration (Goodman 2007). This last phase coincides with the backlash against multiculturalism that recently has swept through Europe. Partly in reaction to this heightened public awareness, the city of Bremen established a "Council for Integration" as an advising body to provide guidance with respect to questions about integrating the city's migrants. The two main German parties—the Social Democrats and Christian Democrats—both consider the Council to be the only legitimate representative of migrants, whereas the Green Party criticizes this political body's dependence on, if not outright control through the Senate. Migrants do take part in this Council—most of them are employees in charity organizations (*Wohlfahrtsverbänden*) and migrant associations.

In contrast to the more civil society-based migrant movements and organizations of the 1980s and early 1990s, the Council has almost entirely refrained from advocating political demands. In addition, the state-monitored and controlled Council[6] has diminished the role of independent migrant associations. The funding policy and the Senate's decision to stop institutional support for migrant associations, without substitution, resulted in a weakening of these associations' organizational resources. The main reason for ending this formerly important funding scheme was, according to an interviewee from the Department of Immigration (*Referat für Zuwanderung*), the danger of exclusion. This agency, whose portfolio addresses the situation of migrants, generally argues that the institutional support of migrant associations is not part of its mandate:

> Most of the time it is like this: they are stuck in those associations forever, they cannot leave them … The question is: should more migrant associations also be funded by us so that more withdrawal happens? … So it cannot be our interest

6 These findings refer to data collection which took place between 2005–2006. As of 2009, when the Councils' former German chairman, an employee of the senate was replaced with a committee of migrants, state control was decisively reduced and the Council slowly started to advocate for political goals.

> that [migrants] do something for themselves in their secluded associations.[7] (Member of the Integration Office, Bremen, 2006)

According to members of the Senate, the only initiatives from migrants that are deemed worthy of funding are those that promote mainstream institutions in politics and civil society. In contrast, attempts to maintain or strengthen a group's cultural or religious identity are seen as illegitimate and at odds with the goals of this political authority in the city:

> Ok, they should meet each other and nurture their culture—that's ok with me. However, we do not need to subsidize this with state funding. They can do whatever they want and if they have an interest, if they think that this is important for their identity, they should pay for it by themselves.[8] (Member of the Integration Office, Bremen, 2006)

This rejection of institutional funding with reference to the allegedly alienating fostering of ethno-cultural identities is also directed against parents' associations. Although these migrant-initiated associations are designed to promote the integration of migrants' children into the German school system, they also fall under the generalized suspicion that they nourish social disintegration and radicalism among particular ethnic groups. The argument is that these groups would retreat from the public sphere by holding meetings in their neighborhoods instead of in the classrooms.

Our interviews with political decision-makers in Bremen point persistently to the central policy that migrant associations should not receive any institutional funding. The arguments used in this frame refer to a concept of integration that rejects the idea of independent political organizations for minorities and political advocacy directed at migrant identities. These arguments have shaped a political climate in which institutional funding for migrant organizations with a former annual budget of €300,000 was scrapped without any substitution. These organizations can now turn only to Bremen's general program for city development, the explicit goal of which is to strengthen local engagement in order to avoid the disintegration of local society.

Our interviews from Leipzig revealed an even stronger rejection of institutional support for migrants. As migrant and pro-migrant organizations in Leipzig were all founded after German unification in 1990, their experience and history radically differs from that of similar organizations in Bremen. Many associations are run by volunteers or job-holders on temporary, hence unsustainable work schemes (*Arbeitsbeschaffungsmaßnahmen*). Rather than claiming rights from the receiving society, migrant organizations in Leipzig commonly address their claims on the migrant communities. Representatives encourage their members to adapt to

7 Translation by authors; Bremen 2007.

8 Translation by authors; Bremen 2007.

the German system by referring to its high quality as compared to health care systems in the homeland. Therefore, barriers faced by migrants attempting to access the local health care system are often not perceived by the latter and their representatives.

Claim-making voices that are heard are often those with a prominent status or a favorable political position in the city, such as the Commissioner of Foreigner Affairs or pro-migrant associations that work on a regional level. Officially, 20 (pro-)migrant associations were established in Leipzig in addition to the 22 intercultural associations and several religious associations, unofficial networks and projects that deal with migrants.[9]

Most migrant associations at the regional and city level could be categorized as self-help groups that are based on voluntary support structures and hardly funded. Their members aim to increase migrants' inclusion in the host society by promoting institutional and labor market access, as well as by providing housing and health care assistance, legal support, information about state institutions and language training. The regional association for Foreign-Citizens in Saxonia was founded in 1993 and limits its activities to the larger cities, including Leipzig. This is similar to the regional organization, RAA (Regional Office for Questions of Foreigners and Ethnic German Migrants/SALVE), which opened a branch in Leipzig in 2005. Importantly, both associations mainly target asylum-seekers, refugees and in the case of RAA/SALVE, ethnic Germans, while citizens with a background of migration are not considered vulnerable.

An exclusively Leipzig-based migrant association founded in 1994 similarly focuses on integration issues by targeting Jewish settlers and migrants from the former Soviet Union. In line with this, a group of Vietnamese migrants established an Association for Vietnamese women[10] which, since its formal institutionalization in 2000, receives city funding for a full position.

The case studies revealed a striking contrast between national policies directed toward the promotion of migrant identities and regional/city policies that reject these national endeavors. On the city level we find varying degrees of effort to undermine migrants' institutionalization and homeland-oriented identity formation processes. By developing participatory patterns over a period of three decades of activism, migrants in Bremen managed to nevertheless participate indirectly in the policy-making process. Meanwhile, migrants in Leipzig, have a much shorter history of civil engagement as 70 percent of them only arrived in the mid 1990s. They hardly involve themselves in the policy or political process and mainly remain on the self-help level with little contact to government policy-making.

9 This includes the organization of intercultural events.

10 Verein Vietnamesischer Frauen in Leipzig e.V.

Migrants' Participation in Italian Public Life: The Dominance of Non-Migrant Civil Society Organizations

In Italy, the issue of migrant participation in public life has been widely discussed (Bozzini and Fella 2008). This discussion has above all been with regard to the way in which regularly resident migrants should be granted citizenship and the right to vote, and the timescale regarding such a process. However, no other types of participation have been central to debates in the public sphere and no proposals to encourage participation have been successful enough to become part of the parliamentary record.

The Italian law regarding citizenship dates back to 1992 (Law 'New Norms on Citizenship' of 5 February 1992 published in the Official Gazette n. 38 of 15-2-1992) and is characterized by a complex, long and uncertain procedure which leaves aspiring migrants in a state of uncertainty and disenfranchised status that limits their willingness to participate (and its effectiveness). Discretionary factors considered in granting citizenship can include the general conduct of migrants during their period of residence, their level of integration in Italian society, income, fulfillment of fiscal obligations and the judgment of the applicant's willingness to become member of the Italian nation. These factors have a discouraging impact on political participation.

The immigration law (Turco-Napolitano Law, 1998) supported the right of foreigners legally living in Italy to participate in local public life, particularly for those having a residency card. The law only allows participation in associations and trade union activities, however, and foresees the creation of consulting bodies at national, regional and local level. By the end of the 1980s, many associations promoted by the migrants themselves (based on national, ethnic and religious belonging) had been formed. However, they tend to be weak, fragmented, small-scale and non-professional, devoting their energies to cultural initiatives rather than political mobilization (Caritas 2010; Zincone 2001, 2006). Even if alliances among migrant associations have been formed in recent years (for instance *Comitato Immigrati in Italia* and *Forum delle Comunità Straniere in Italia-FOCSVI*), most migrant associations are committed to supply identity and solidarity resources to its members. Many of the associations are transnationally organized and have a homeland bias, whereas other mixed or local associations are more oriented toward dialogue with social and institutional actors in Italy (Allasino et al. 1995; Palidda and Consoli 2005). In terms of rights promotion, associations led by white Italians without a background of migration dominate, particularly those linked to trade unions and the Catholic Church. The general result of this is a situation that one can define as "white anti-racism" (that is activism in the field being dominated by white Italians).

The ethos of the Turco-Napolitano law was one of cautious incorporation, not only providing avenues for the expression of migrants' interests in the public sphere, but also for the repression of irregular immigration. The repressive element was augmented in a successive law, the Bossi-Fini, which defined migrants mainly in terms of their role as workers and increased provisions for their expulsion when their role in the job market ceases. Residence papers now last for half of the time they used to and family rejoining is severely restricted. This move increased all elements of uncertainty and therefore undermined the assertion of migrants' presence in the political and the public spheres, making their associations appear less relevant since incorporation was now defined in much narrower terms. The Bossi-Fini law marked a transition to a new right-wing government that was elected in 2001 and re-elected in 2008, thus providing *de facto* continuity to an increasing perception of migrants as an unwanted cultural and security threat. Nonetheless, several migrant associations funded at the beginning of migration flows to Italy in the 1980s have survived.

The Italian associations that have flowered in this sector since the 1980s are of a varied nature. Many fill the void created by the absence of an organized institutional response to immigration and thus find themselves on the front-lines of service provision and assistance for new migrant arrivals. Associations receive funds from a variety of sources. Some collect funds from the resident ethnic community. Several receive varying levels of support from City Councils. Occasionally they receive funds or resources from the Catholic Church or from generalist associations.

Associations perform a variety of functions which include providing information points for migrants, offering cultural and linguistic mediation, managing social integration projects, providing assistance in finding accommodation and work and offering literacy and professional training. They have also been involved in promoting religious and cultural understanding, assisting in the regularization of migrants, acting as advocates for migrant rights and sometimes taking part in consultative bodies with various levels of government. Different strategies have been adopted to tackle the problems facing migrants, ranging from collaboration with institutions in order to ameliorate the everyday hardships migrants suffer, to a more intransigent social opposition to the role institutions play in exacerbating the problems faced by migrants. While strategies differ, the dignity and rights of migrants remain paramount concerns for all associations operating in the field, bringing many of them together in alliances to challenge racism and prejudice and raise awareness of the problems facing migrants. Nevertheless, scarcity of resources, difference in strategies and priorities and an immersion in the every-day problems facing migrants on the part of many local associations have placed limits on the ability of associations to form a broader and cohesive antiracist civil society front. Since the advent of the center-right government in 2001 and its subsequent re-election in 2008, the closed nature of the political system toward these associations has further weakened their advocacy role, contributing to a climate of pessimism in pro-migrant civil society (Geddes 2008).

Among the measures aimed at promoting the integration of foreigners, the center-left government (1996–2001) had instituted some national representation bodies and had reorganized those which already existed but had never performed their duties steadily: a Commission for the Integration of Immigrants; a National

Fund for Migration Policies; a Consultative Committee for Immigrants involving the various associations that work with migrants in deliberative discussions on the problems they face; and a National Coordination Body. By 2001, these bodies were still not working properly. Under the first center-right government (2001–2008), decision-makers in Italy tended to view the control of immigration in functional and legalist terms, not leaving much space for the construction of positive and efficient integration policies. This climate has continued and even radicalized in the last center-right government since 2008. Support for the equitable inclusion of migrants into public life and for the fight against discrimination and racism is generally absent, as is the presence of interlocutors open to dialogue within the government. Where meetings do take place, they do not last very long and civil society organizations see them as deprived of any intention of real consultation. Consultations are rare (both for associations and trade unions), taking place only informally and for addressing specific situations. They depend on the personal rapport between association representatives and select decision-makers and bureaucrats in government ministries.

Among the measures aimed at promoting the integration of foreigners, the center-left government (1996–2001) had also instituted or reinforced some local representation bodies, such as the Consultative Committees of Immigrants, at the regional, provincial and municipal level. Concerning the municipal level, however, data gathered by the Study Center of International Politics (CESPI 2002) shows that in December 2002, few Italian municipalities had instruments of political participation for foreigners.[11] Various research on their functioning also points out that the level of their representativeness is limited (Zincone 2006) due to factors such as the weakness of associations, the fact that associations have to be registered with the Department of Social Affairs of the Presidency of the Council of Ministers and, more generally, the ambiguity of the norms regarding such representation (Fieri 2005). This situation has not improved in recent years.

At the local level, the Consultative Committee is not influential and it does not take part in the meetings of the town council. This possibility is only accorded to its chairperson—many times only if invited and always without the right to vote. The power of local Consultative Committees can range from the possibility to express opinions when asked by local administration to the possibility of expressing an opinion even if not mandatory. Moreover, opinions can be expressed on all of the issues or only on those regarding immigration. As far as the designation of the members is concerned, usually the norms request the participation of at least two migrant associations' representatives but do not specify a clear procedure on how to choose them. *Choosing individuals that are really representative of*

11 In the survey, 12.4 percent of the municipalities considered had instituted a consultative committee or an immigrants' council, whereas only 2.8 percent had provided the presence of an added councilor. The latter seems to be the preferred solution of provincial capitals and towns of the center and south of Italy, while consultative committees are more frequent in the north.

communities appears to be the main problem: Sometimes there are two or more associations of citizens from the same country, or there are cultural associations of citizens from different countries, assuming their shared national 'cultures' (for example: Albania, Macedonia and Kosovo).

Locally, the choice of representatives is often done through co-optation by local authorities on the basis of the size of the communities or their political participation (Fieri 2005). Only in very few cases do local consultative bodies provide the eligibility of foreign members, as in the case of "Added Councilors at a municipal level (one or more, according to the size of the Commune) and of "Elective Consultative Committees" at a municipal and provincial level. As foreign members are never the majority, *Italian associations assume leadership within these bodies*. Public institutions often seem to prefer the mediation of the Italian pro-migrant associations rather than the direct participation of migrants themselves (Caritas Italiana 2010).

Conclusions

The involvement of migrant and minority associations in politics in general, and policy arenas in particular reflects structural and cultural opportunities for these civil society institutions to make their voice heard. In all of our national case studies there is a general recognition of the role that political participation plays in the successful integration of migrants. While in the European context the EU might be the most active actor in promoting steps toward enhancing opportunities for migrants' political participation (see Council of Europe 1992 and 1999), the concept of migrants' political engagement has received widespread endorsement. Additionally, in Western democracies there is a tendency in current governance configurations that applies to all three of our national case studies: Contemporary public administrations have shown an increasing degree of dependence on and willingness to collaborate with civil society actors that provide them with information, guidance and, most critically, legitimacy. For a variety of reasons, governance in contemporary Western democracies is increasingly reliant on the inclusion of non-governmental associations in the policy process. Against this backdrop, new forms of NGOs' involvement in the formation and implementation of public policy have emerged.

At the same time, there are notable differences in how this process has evolved and been institutionalized in the three national contexts under investigation. Given distinct political and cultural traditions in Canada, Germany and Italy, migrant associations are present in public-political life to different degrees and in different forms. Applied to our schematic summary our three cases about the continuum of migrants gaining voice as loosely organized citizens' to migrants formally included in the policy process as follows:

Table 2.2 Degrees of migrants' involvement with policy process compared

Intersection with policy process
No involvement in policy process ↓↓ ↓ **ITALY** ↓**GERMANY** ↓ ↓**CANADA** ↓↓ **High degree of involvement in policy process**

Most notably, the Canadian case is distinct with regard to how deeply entrenched and institutionalized the representation of migrant and minority associations is. Meanwhile in Germany and Italy, these associations have only recently gained visibility and significance in the public and policy-making arenas. They have become far more firmly part of the public administration environment and routinized processes of community consultation in Canada. The following chapter will investigate how these national contexts shape and provide opportunities for migrant associations in the health care sector.

Particularly in our European case studies, our analysis also indicates the emergence of a generalized trend: While there is a more distinct emphasis on integration and political inclusion of migrants, in recent years there has also been a decisive turn in public opinion and in the political establishment away from a multiculturalist ethos. This reaction might be stronger on the right than on the left, but appears to embrace all political divides and therefore shapes the prospects of all migrant associations (which are losing legitimacy and gradually coming to be seen as an obstacle to integration). Their presence would simply solidify pre-existing identities and hinder processes of integration. Possibly as a reaction to decreasing legitimacy and resources, mainly for lack of funding many migrants seem to abandon associational forms as an avenue of claim-making, and alternatively emphasize religious affiliations and forms of religious aggregations that are less dependent on state resources and legitimacy, as the Bremen trend from associations to mosques and Pentecostal Churches seem to paradigmatically exemplify. The situation is similar in Italy, where the current right-wing government has closed many consultative institutions and embraced an anti-multiculturalist ethos that does not facilitate efforts at establishing a viable presence of migrant organizations in civil society. In turn, the Italian left has been an articulate and political advocate for migrants' and minorities' rights. However, this form of political advocacy is very much based on established church or civil society-based organizations in which migrants themselves only play a very marginal role.

A separate set of considerations apply to Canada. If on the one hand a similar reaction to multiculturalism is increasingly also manifest in Canada, on the other hand this does not easily translate into the closure or undermining of associationism in general and migrant associationism in particular. Unlike in Europe (where associations have often been conceptualized as akin to business interest groups and therefore as the voice of particularist interests which are a potential threat to democracy), within the Anglo-American tradition the Toquevillian thought (of conceiving associations as necessary safeguards against the menace of an overpowering state, as an alternative means of community-based service delivery and as a marker of communities' self-reliance) has persisted. In this context, migrant associations have thus continued to remain relevant.

Our evaluation of the effectiveness of associational representation is based on its overall role at all levels of governance. This is mainly determined by the size of the sector, its resource base and organizational effectiveness in service delivery and advocacy. As argued, this varies widely across locations but there are identifiable national trends. Thus the demonstrated weakness of Italian associational representation in Naples is hardly compensating by the more effective civil society in Trento.

However, one must of course also contextualize the interaction between associational representation and health institutions in relation to other social and political structures providing an avenue for expressions of organized migrant interests. If we proceed with this contextualization we will then be able to more comprehensively document our assertion that there are less effective channels for migrants' voices in Italy and better ones in Germany and better still in Canada on other grounds as well. While an all-inclusive analysis of the features that make migrants' voices effective would be very wide-ranging here we would like to point to three aspects: (1) the structure of organized civil society; (2) its relation with agonistic arenas; and (3) its relation with processes of opinion formation in society.

As for the first aspect (1), it should be noted that one cannot simply discuss the role of civil society without reference to its composition, organizational structures and power bases. In policy terms an effective civil society could be configured as a strong decision-shaping impact of narrow elites or broader societal processes of consensus aggregation of its multiple actors. Its organizations can be more or less internally democratic and this will also result in different configurations of the sector. We posit that an effective inclusion of civil society is one that provides channels for deliberation in which organized interests do not represent the voices of oligarchies but authentic processes of consensus aggregation. In order to do so organizations have to provide internal spaces for deliberation and need to acquire a presence in external deliberating structures (Mendelberg 2002). This, in our case studies, does not typically happen in the Italian case due to the fact that organized civil society tends to be represented by generalist indigenous associational actors thereby hindering channels of deliberation. In addition, migrants' voices are muted by the relative fragmentation of the Italian migrant population which is poorly organized in small constituencies of nationalities whose contacts are hindered by linguistic, religious and cultural differences. This again favors the emergence of oligarchies of self-interested actors sometimes merely interested in the particularistic appropriation of public funds.

Secondly (2), migrants' functional representation should be framed in relation to other forms of social and political representation as it complements and influences them. Thus, it is alternative to representation in agonistic arenas, but its functions are influenced by what happened in these arenas and how these arenas are structured. A full analysis of the relation between functional representation and electoral representation is not possible here but we have examined some aspects that could now be usefully contextualized. An aspect that we examined in our analysis is the relation between functional representation and electoral laws. In Italy then at national level the current electoral law does not provide a selection of the representatives by the electorate. It is based on blocked lists selected by the parties. This gives a disproportionate power to party apparatuses which has an impact on how civil society associations are selected for policy inclusion and resourcing. There is then a deficit of electoral representation which is compounded by the weakness and biased character of national-level associational representation described in the previous paragraphs. Given the centralized nature of the Italian state and the related primacy of national level politics, it is also for this reason then that the Italian case is conceptualized as unable to channel the views of migrants to the policy-making machinery. In addition, a majoritarian system is typically less open to functional representation of small constituencies such as migrants than one based on proportional laws. Italy made a transition to a majoritarian system in which as previously argued the ruling parties are ideologically unreceptive to migrants' advocacy. This is different from the federal nature of the German state in which there is a proportional electoral law and in which substantial autonomy and resources are controlled at local level. The same consideration also applies to Canada which includes both an effective federal architecture and inclusive electoral laws at all levels of governance.

Thirdly (3), to the extent that the effectiveness of civil society is in part based on its size which in turn is related to social capital, we need to factor in different cross-national distributions of social capital, particularly of the bridging type. Again in this perspective the relative disadvantage of Italy emerges clearly (Wallace and Pichler 2007). A broader and effective civil society sector will improve the availability of volunteers for health-related donations of time and energy and therefore also the entire service delivery aspect of migrants' health, as we will see in the following chapter. In terms of the advocacy function of civil society, one needs to relay not only on the amount of voluntarism available in a society but on an informed population able and ready to engage in deliberative processes. A non-oligarchic civil society needs then an educated and informed population and in turn an open public sphere based on non-monopolistic processes of opinion formation. This calls into question the role of the media, which are increasingly becoming a crucial aspect of effective social citizenship (Urbinati 2006). From this point of view monopolistic processes in Italian media ownership over several decades have hindered the effectiveness of public deliberation and negatively impacted the advocacy potential of Italian civil society. This has happened to a far less extent in Canada or Germany.

Chapter 3
Political Advocacy in the Health Care System

Introduction: Participation in the Field of Health Care

In this chapter, we will shift our focus from migrant associations in general to the specific role these associations play in the health field. In this context, the interviews and the analysis of the documents are aimed at examining the different modalities of participation in the health sector in Canada, Germany, and Italy. In particular, in this chapter we introduce the main actors (migrant associations/ pro-migrant associations/ ethnic communities/ public authorities/ insurance companies/ and so on) that participate in health-related policy-making in the three countries. We provide an exploration of agenda-setting processes, that is: who decides which issues are discussed in the structured processes of participation; which are the strategies and the institutional practices adopted in the health systems in order to institutionalize the interests of migrants in the policy-making process (the types of engagement and its formalization); how requests for participation in the policy-making process by associations are expressed and the responsiveness of decision-makers; which kind of requests groups put forward; the purpose of participation; the sense of identification with the issues frequently raised among migrants; the presence and the mobilization of ethnic groups with a specific social capital; the presence of networks among the subjects interested in the issue; and which relationships exist among associations and between activists and public organizations.

First, some general considerations are useful for defining health as a policy sector. The concept of health, since the Alma-Ata Conference[1] (WHO 1978), has been revisited substantially. It is now defined as a more complex cultural frame that is linked not only to the actual health characteristics of individuals, but also to interpretations of how health is socially represented and to the environmental and social factors that determine it—a cluster of factors which are then psychological,

1 At the international level, the right to health is recognized in the Universal Declaration of Human Rights adopted by the General Assembly of the United Nations in 1948 (where in article 25 it is established that "Everyone has the right to a standard of living adequate for the health and well-being of himself and of his family, including food, clothing, housing and medical care and necessary social services …"), as well as by various other international dispositions such as the International Covenant on Economic, Social and Cultural Rights (signed in 1966) and the Declaration of Alma-Ata of 1978.

social and physiological (Ingrosso 2006; Maturo 2004). Health is no longer considered to be something that you lose or gain at a specific point in time, but rather the result of a long and complex path. Therefore, it is now understood that health policies do not just consist of resources to be distributed or services to be offered. In Western countries, there is a tendency to modify the way health is managed and organized and to adopt a more complex perspective in the health sector—a more flexible and adaptable approach that takes into account the plurality of actors and seeks to aggregate their diverse experiences and competences. On the one hand, due to the difficulties of measuring needs exclusively through technical surveys and managerial tools, the need to *involve citizens* in the construction of health policies has become increasingly clearer. On the other hand, the need emerges to offer more articulate *services to customers*, where health assistance must be integrated and coordinated with other types of interventions. The general trend, therefore, is to create integrated policies; that is, to face issues from different perspectives by overcoming the separation among competences and sectors. In order to achieve this goal, however, it is necessary to be clear about what strategies of citizen involvement and service delivery are put in place in different locations, their effectiveness, and in this context, examine the role of associations.

In assessing the role of migrants' groups in the health field, we then need a set of recognized standards with regard to what functions they can exert in principle. On this basis, we can examine our case studies and assess them in terms of a set of ideal standards. As has already been briefly discussed in the previous chapter, these standards are provided by the literature on migrant groups, and on the functions of civil society in policy-making and service delivery arenas more generally. Once the roles that migrant and pro-migrant civil society organizations can play in activities of policy-making are clarified, it will be possible to assess their specific performance in our case studies.

In this chapter, we will specifically examine three general types of functions. First, civil society organizations can provide *information* to the policy process. Citizens' involvement presumes that their competence is valued and their knowledge is channeled into the policy process. Second, citizens' *advocacy efforts* have to be valued, particularly when they address problematic issues and react to unsatisfactory situations. Public services and political structures need to be able to respond constructively to the advocacy efforts of sectors of the population, such as migrants, whose needs are arguably not satisfactorily attended. Third, if good *service delivery* requires the integration of policies (that is, the ability of public services to face issues from different perspectives), an ability to form alliances with other social and political actors is required in order to improve service delivery. This third function also encompasses aspects of the other two. In this sense, a role frequently attributed to civil society groups becomes a support in guaranteeing the high quality of policies. This implies a set of distinctive contributions to policy formation, implementation and monitoring on the one hand, and to policy delivery on the other. The two aspects are interconnected, as in terms of the first goal (policy effectiveness) they can redress (at least to some extent) the sometimes insufficient legitimacy of policy-making institutions (in the eyes of particular social constituencies, such as migrants) by increasing legitimacy through effective policy delivery. On the basis of these ideal standards, we will now examine our national cases to test which of these goals are accomplished and which are the blockages to a more effective role for migrants' organizations. The following paragraphs will therefore first introduce how the issue of migration has typically been processed in the national context of our case studies. They will then consider the three areas of knowledge brokerage, advocacy functions and service delivery functions in the respective two cities that have been identified for in-depth analysis in each of the national contexts.

Participation in Health: The Case of Canada

As elaborated in the previous chapter, the political and institutional context for migrants' engagement and advocacy in the health care sector in Canada differs considerably from our European case studies. While in Germany, and in particular in Italy, the political voice of migrants is a relatively new phenomenon, it is a legacy of Canadian multiculturalism to have encouraged migrant organizations and community groups to articulate the concerns of their clientele in the public arena. Beyond the general commitment to publicly endorsing diversity and promoting equal opportunities, Canadian-style multiculturalism has established a set of expectations about good governance that the health care system cannot avoid to respond to.

Functions and Limits of Canadian Civil Society in Health Care

One key element that shapes the Canadian context in this respect is how to translate the normative expectations of multiculturalism into effective modes of governance. It is very much part of the legacy of Canadian multiculturalism since its inception in the early 1970s that the consultation with and the input from the community have developed into key components of what the status of cultural diversity and minorities in society should be. In this respect, community engagement is widely seen to be an integral part of managing cultural diversity. The health care sector as a central area of public policy-making is not exempt from this expectation. The Community Engagement Department of Vancouver Coastal Health declared programmatically in 2005:

> VCH recognizes that community engagement is part of good decision-making processes. With such diverse communities in the region, having a formalized approach for gathering feedback from the public is vital to our organization … VCH staff actively consult clients, patients, residents and other community stakeholders to improve decisions and ensure that the system is responsive to their concerns. (VCH 2005: 1)

Good decision-making refers to both the legitimacy of the process and effectiveness of its outcomes. The latter aspect speaks to the second fundamental dynamic that encourages modes of incorporating migrant representatives more thoroughly into governance structures. It has to do with the very mode in which health care provision operates: in particular in major urban centers migrant and minority communities constitute an increasingly important clientele for health care providers. Health care services need to reflect the specific needs of these groups. The term 'responsiveness' indicates this fundamental concern about appropriate care for clients that the health care system needs to take into consideration as a state-managed service provider. It is telling how a representative from the Ministry and Health Authority reflects on where incentives and initiatives for community engagement come from. Our interviewees rarely refer to any fixed procedural rules but to how the interaction with the community emerges almost naturally out of what the health care sector does on a daily basis:

> hmm// that, you know, it's not something that the organization has said. I mean, they do say that all the time, right? You do need to have community linkages, but nobody sits around to me and says, 'You must develop community linkages.' You know, like, … / it's because we know that's important and we go out and do it. (Ministry and Health Authority representative, Vancouver, 2006)

Community engagement is described as an integral part of health care's routine mode of operation. A critical component in this process is the seemingly mundane, albeit critical collection of accurate information about the clientele that is being served.

> And the lovely thing is that VCH, and Mental Health Services are open enough to want that information—they want programs improved for immigrant communities. They want the programs running at the optimum not only for English-speakers, but for non-English speakers. (Ministry and Health Authority representative, Vancouver, 2006)

> On the other hand, there has never been in Quebec a complete acceptance of the immigrant population as being a target population that needs to be addressed very specifically. In other words, ACCÉSSS[2] has always been saying that the diversity of a population has to be accounted for when you provide services. And that has not been the general approach. (Migrant Association, Montreal, 2006)

Our interviews show that community engagement is also instrumental for related aspects of information collection and dissemination: It is said to raise awareness of migrants' needs in the health care sector (educating staff), to disseminate the

2 *Alliance des communautés culturelles pour l'égalité dans la santé et les services sociaux*, see Chapter 5 for more details on this organization.

information on existing services for these groups in the community, and to set the agenda for institutional reform. In this perspective, community engagement is regularly described by staff in the health care sector as 'mutually beneficial' for service providers and community groups.

However, considering how community engagement is to some degree inscribed into the functional imperatives of the health care sector, it is worth noting that there is also an institutionally ingrained tendency to keep this engagement to a minimum. This becomes manifest in the following reflection on the scope of community engagement from the perspective of a representative from a health authority:

> because I was reading through the VIHA community engagement strategy and everything is 'if time and resources allow it, we will talk to people, but it's very expensive, so we'll be very selective in our community engagement.' ... So it wasn't that it was a big priority of the organization. It was, it felt like they had to do that for accountability purposes, but it was a very reluctant approach, whereas it seems, ... that, and, do you find that there's, that the board of, of Vancouver Coastal is very committed to the community engagement or is it like, OK. (Ministry and Health Authority representative, Vancouver, 2006)

While serving the needs of customers, community engagement is a labor-intensive and costly undertaking. The interaction and exchange with the community can also be perceived to put undue pressure on limited resources in the system.

What emerges in the Canadian context is an—at times—reluctant acceptance of the health care sector to endorse community engagement as an important feature of how it operates and relates to the social groups that it serves. On the one hand, there is the publicly and politically endorsed claim that community engagement should be part of good and accountable forms of governance and that health care provision can be organized more effectively if the community gains a voice in the process of deliberation and decision-making. On the other hand, there is a manifest moment of institutional inertia. Community engagement requires time and resources; it cannot rely on a well-established institutional framework for incorporating civil society actors.

Engagement and Advocacy: Different Models in Montreal and Vancouver

Still, while there are nationally-specific features of how migrants find a public "voice" in the Canadian case, there is considerable variation in how issues related to health care provisions are articulated and negotiated in different regional or even local contexts. One could make a valid argument that it is indeed the absence of proper resources and institutional means that accounts for the variation in scope and form of community engagement in the health care sector. A representative of an influential migrant organization from Montreal, describes the variation in terms of the influence of community actors as follows:

> In some case, because you have a few that are very strong leaders, or traditionally come from a community where there is a tradition, they will, eventually be in positions of being advisors or leaders, being elected to boards, being elected to committees. But this is like sporadic. Again the major stumbling block is that the whole thing is so haphazard, that in terms of funding for community organizations, in terms of participation on boards, committees, or in terms of being able to serve a population, you got everything there. You got some very good situations, some middle of the road and some real horror stories. So, you got a whole spectrum of possible answers, and it's all left to local people to somehow organize themselves to get the service that they need. (Migrant Association, Montreal, 2006)

There clearly is the decisive role of local leadership and the volatile funding situation that shape the engagement and influence of civil society organizations in the health care sector. Yet there are also some more structural features that can help us to understand the variation between our two cities under investigation in Canada. One factor that resurfaced frequently in our study is the degree to which an ethno-cultural community is well established and has developed modes of articulating its claims in the public and political arena. It is the "community" itself that is diverse with respect to how much recognition and influence individual migrant and minority groups have.

> Then what has happened is over the years, depending on the arrival of different groups, some of them did manage to create some kind of health care structure, some private, some public and some para-public, but over the years the new arrivals, the people who have arrived in the last fifteen, twenty years, did not have that opportunity, have not had the opportunity to create their own structures that help the people in their own community. … So there is an enormous spectrum there, from people who are well served to people who are not served at all. So there's quite a … you have to consider that there is something like around 160 different ethnic groups in Quebec. (Migrant Association, Montreal, 2006)

The strength and organizational resources of migrant organizations are also likely to be a factor in how our two cities in Canada, Montreal and Vancouver, have established distinct institutional routines and legal frameworks to organize community engagement in the health care sector. Both provinces, Quebec and British Columbia, introduced channels through which the interests of cultural communities are integrated into the policy process, albeit through two different models: In Quebec we have a consultative structure at the ministerial level which allows migrant groups to gain direct access to the Minister of Health. In British Columbia there is a more decentralized engagement framework in place, which helps to collect and articulate the concerns of different communities. The first model is driven by an initiative of the Ministry itself while the second is fuelled primarily by a bottom-up process organized by civil society groups. Surely, we note that people have been involved in more ad-hoc engagement that also shapes the practices in health care service delivery. Still, both models have established an important institutional mode to channel communication and to deal with disputes that, as we will see in greater detail in Chapter 5, have an important effect on how political advocacy unfolds in both cities and how effective the respective strategies of community engagement are.

The strategy for involving migrants' concerns in the health care system in Quebec resulted in the formation of a provincial committee in 2004 (Provincial Committee on the Dispensation of Services to Persons from Ethnic and Cultural Communities) designed to advise the Minister of Health and Social Services on the claims of migrant and minority groups. The committee provides advice on matters concerning the health and social services network with particular focus on the needs of migrant communities. The committee consists of a dozen people named by the Minister who were nominated by various migrant communities and come from different regions of the province.

In contrast to Quebec, in British Columbia the strategy utilized for involving migrants' concerns in the policy framework is through a Community Engagement Framework. Since 2002, Vancouver Coastal Health (VCH) has proceeded with consulting communities via community health advisory committees that work on a whole range of health-related themes. Moreover, the government allocated SMART (Sharon Martin Community Health Fund)[3] funds for promoting community capacity building.

Effectiveness of Community Engagement and Political Advocacy

The creation and composition of these two models of community engagement reflect an acknowledgement of the need for structures that allow for migrant and minority communities to voice their concern and, to some degree, be included in the consultation and decision-making process. However, the effectiveness of both models within the particular urban context in Montreal and Vancouver respectively is difficult to detect and contested among those who are involved in the community engagement process themselves.

In the case of Quebec, some community groups underline that the formation of a provincial committee has provided them with a legally enshrined entitlement to be in included in the policy process. In this perspective the committee is seen as an important step toward overcoming the relative marginalization and powerlessness that some migrant communities have experienced *vis-à-vis* the policy process and

3 The SMART supports 72 programs in non-profit agencies throughout the Vancouver Coastal Health region that have developed projects geared towards helping people stay healthy in their communities. Established in 1997, the SMART Fund currently provides $3.7 million in annual funding to programs that support members of society who face multiple barriers in accessing health services.

the health care sector. Here is a voice from a migrant association about the value of the committee for advocacy:

> It's in the law, …, and it says that the Minister can decide the composition of the committee and what it should do. That's what our Minister does—he decided what to do and the composition. The Bill was recognized officially, it was voted in the National Assembly, so it has a legal existence. That's very important. So the Minister can tell the committee to give him advice on the delivery of health services and social services for people or ethno-cultural communities.[4] It determines its composition and its rules. So it's a tool that the Minister gave himself to have an ear to cultural communities. Because yes, we say that we are all Canadians, Quebecers, we have programs, … if I am not at ease, the Minister should be aware of it. That's why we have a direct link with him. (Migrant Association, Montreal, 2006)

The legal empowerment and the direct link to the ministerial level of decision-making are considered to be major assets in allowing for an effective community engagement process: "So that's our lobbying function, means that we look, we analyze bills, we analyze *projets de loi*, and we try to then put forward a memoire, briefs, so that when we go to the legislative commissions, parliamentary commission, we can put forward on behalf of cultural communities" (Migrant Association, Montreal, 2006). Yet, this view is challenged by those who see the committee primarily as a token for creating a sense of accountability rather than a genuine vehicle for participation and decision-making. There are doubts about how influential concerns raised in this committee actually are in terms of influencing policy outcomes.

> However, since 2004 I met the Minister only once. I'm not happy with that, we should be meeting the Minister regularly. But only once, he came, he shook hands and left. Since 2004 we've had meetings every two months. We're looking at specific aspects of health care, we're looking at studies that have been made, but so far our influence has been very minimal. Because it goes through the bureaucracy, we inform the secretariat and the secretariat will take our recommendations and it goes to the Sous-Ministre. The Sous-Ministre, then, if he decides that it's worth it he will take it all the way up to the minister. But it's not, we don't have the ear of the minister on a regular basis. There's no direct link to the minister. So it filters. In a bureaucracy it filters from what xxxx said over here, by the time it gets to the Minister, it has been watered-down and wishy-washy. (Migrant Association, Montreal, 2006)

---

4 "Ethno cultural communities" is the official term used for migrant communities of different national or ethnic origin in the Canadian context. Because the term does not differentiate between ethnic or national background, we prefer to use the category "migrant communities" or as in the German context "People with a Migration Background."

The "British Columbia model" is based on a different mode of facilitating community engagement and thus faces different challenges to its effectiveness. Here the core idea is to nourish a more decentralized form on interaction between community associations, the health service organizations and political authorities. Opportunities to voice the concerns of diverse communities materialize in a variety of often community-based projects that engage political authorities or health care providers. A prominent example is the Multicultural Health Fair that is organized annually by the Affiliation of Multicultural Societies and Service Agencies (AMSSA) in Vancouver (the largest event of its kind in Canada; similar fairs have recently been set up in smaller communities across British Columbia).

> The Multicultural Health Fair is another example. We are bringing representatives from the health authorities, community health, the organizations, and our member agencies to attend, but not just attend the fair, have a nice time and leave. The next day there is a 3 hour workshop that will be about developing a fair, who you work with, how you bring it together, and for them to network with each other, network with our steering committee from here, and to develop their own action plans for their own health fair … (Migrant Association, Vancouver, 2006)

There are a couple of significant elements in the way a representative from a migrant association describes this event; it reflects a more general dynamic in how community engagement unfolds in Vancouver: First, the event is initiated by migrant associations; it is a grass-root initiative based on needs articulated in the community. Second, the Multicultural Health Fair creates a cross-sectional form of collaboration between community associations and service providers which allows for mutual learning and the transfer of knowledge into institutional practices in the health care institutions. Thirdly, it promises to create a more sustainable forum for exchange and collaboration through which concerns of diverse communities can be channeled, more community groups be involved, and new initiatives be developed.

At the same time, in this "model" there is no direct institutional arrangement for linking these initiatives to the policy process. It is a far more decentralized and informal process of articulating the concerns of diverse communities and bringing them to the attention of political authorities than in the case of Montreal. The following citation from one of our interviews addresses the status of the networks of collaboration created by AMSSA as an umbrella organization from the perspective of VCH. Here reference is made to a committee on migrant health issues organized by AMSSA. Asked about the form of collaboration the interviewee responded:

> I'd say it's informal. I mean, the committee is formal in the sense that it's an official committee of AMSSA, and we officially, and we pay membership dues, and we attend the committee, um, so no, I guess that makes it formal. (Ministry and Health Authority representative, Vancouver, 2006)

The uncertainty about the status of the committee reflects a general feature of the situation of community engagement in Vancouver: What we find here is a very energetic network of collaborations and initiatives that, however, lack the formalized structure and direct link to political authority as institutionalized by the committee in Montreal. In the subsequent two chapters we will discuss in greater detail what these basic structures mean for addressing issues of access to services and promoting change in the health care system.

Participation in Health Care: The Case of Germany

As already mentioned, research in Germany has revealed remarkable variations between the federal, regional and city level when it comes to migration-related policies and structures. In Germany, civic engagement in the area of migration and health basically started in the 1980s and, while steadily gaining significance, has contributed to the fact that some structures in the German health care system start opening up toward migrants. Awareness of the challenges posed by cultural diversity has replaced a neglectful approach (in which diversity is not relevant for the provision of health care services) to the issue. Activism was dominantly triggered by influential medical directors who, confronted with migrants' access barriers, brought the issue into the public arena via research, conferences and publications. Importantly, health experts from the second generation of migrants are entering the medical field as health care professionals and have contributed to the public discourse since the 1990s by providing at least 50 percent of the activists. Similar to the Health Committee in Quebec, the federal working group Migration and Public Health[5] (founded in 1994 and based in the Ministry of Health) represents the issue of migration and health on the national level. Unlike Quebec's committee, however, the working group neither *represents* the dominant "migrant communities," nor reports to the Minister of Health. It is a loose group consisting of public health experts from health-related state institutions (some of which have a background of migration), the field of science and the policy-making community in all federal states. The working group does not directly advise the ministry, but has prominently contributed to changes in the health care system which resulted in more migrant-friendly health care structures.[6]

In addition, policy deliberations at the national level also include non-state professional medical associations that deal with the issues. These organizations mainly focus on internal professional exchanges during conferences, but are also partly involved in the policy process during public forums with policy-

5 Bundesarbeitskreis Migration und Öffentliche Gesundheit.

6 By migrant-friendly health care structures we are referring to structures that improve migrants' access to health care. These structures could be translation services, cultural mediators, health staff with a migration background, diversity training for health staff, visitor rooms, migrant-specific food offers, multi-religious rooms etc.

makers. Many of these associations are migrant associations. Yet, their role in the decision-making process is limited. As the highest body in the German health care system, the national committee (*Gemeinsamer Bundesausschuß*) determines which services are paid for by the statutory health insurances. Members of this committee show very little interest in the accommodation of migrants' needs, as admitted in the following interview: "The influence of migrants in the committee dealing with national issues is barely possible because we deal with medical supply and not with information for guidelines" (head of the committee dealing with national issues 2006, Berlin). Rather than considering the issue of migration as part of the issue of health, the committee understands its task exclusively in health terms, denying a link with the issue of migration or the importance of migrant-friendly services.

When it comes to the regional and city level, the state is hardly visible in Leipzig and is partly involved in Bremen. Here, representatives of the federal migration and public health working group have initiated the establishment of a "department of migration and health" in the bureau of public health with the aim to improve health conditions for asylum seekers, refugees, and ethnic Germans (*Spätaussiedler*) in Bremen. Next to the determination of minimum standards for the accommodation of this group the health program includes a broad offer of medical support. A doctor of the department migration and health of the public health office offers regular medical consultation in the living quarters of the target group. This model, which throughout Germany came to be known as the "Bremer Modell," has addressed some of the access barriers created by the asylum law (*Asylbewerberleistungsgesetz*) passed in 1993 (Lotze 2009; Mohammadzadeh 2004). Though the department basically focuses on migrant-friendly health care for refugees and asylum seekers, it also offers minor services for citizens with a migration background (HIV/AIDS, translation services, multilingual health information brochures). As a result of the department's activities several policy aims were included in the senate's regional integration concept (2007–2011) which explicitly aim at improving migrants' access to health care. Some welfare organizations have implemented national policies addressing migrants on the local level as well. For Bremen, this is the case with the *Arbeiter Wohlfahrt* (AWO or workers welfare organization) and its focus on migrant-friendly nursing homes. An education based welfare association, the *Paritätisches Bildungswerk* (PBW or Equal Representation Educational Institute) supports projects engaging in diversity management such as the *Bremer Forum-Diversity*. Such often short-lived projects also receive funding from the senate. In Leipzig, however, even the welfare organizations have not been involved in building up migrant-friendly structures. There is simply no nationwide, state-monitored strategy to enable the health care system to respond to the challenge of cultural diversity. Rather, individual organizations inside and outside of the health care system have promoted the issue and triggered institutional reforms. Not surprisingly, the results vary considerably according to the local context, the respective strength of the civil society organizations and the institutional opening for change.

Thus, a first general finding is the marginal or absent state involvement and the disparity of commitment among different regional and city authorities in the intercultural aperture of the health care system. After this general introduction on participation in the field of health care in Germany, the following section will focus on health-related migrant activism in the two selected German cities: Leipzig and Bremen.

Functions and Limits of German Civil Society in Health Care

Group formation and engagement

In the German context, a particularly significant role has traditionally been played by migrant organizations within established migrant communities, such the Turkish community (on which we have focused in more detail). However, several of these organizations have traditionally understood their role in somewhat circumscribed terms. *Saglikli Yasa* (live healthy/live in good health), the first health-based movement established by migrants in Bremen in the 1980s, was not involved in claim- or policy-making at all. Its activities were solely directed at building up self-help structures in the Turkish community and its central concerns were: (1) to reduce drug addiction; (2) to strengthen the position of single mothers; (3) to be involved in family reconciliation; and (4) to create awareness about AIDS and STDs.[7] The group developed Turkish language informational materials on basic health issues. Its members exchanged best practices with already established migrant and pro-migrant organizations in other cities and applied them to their "community."

In the 1990s, this group moved from catering to the needs of its own community to a broader form of political engagement that actually contributed to structural changes in the Bremen health care system by promoting the establishment of a center for traumatized refugees.[8] The group also organized a conference on mental health issues that was partly financed by the regional state. A central aspect of *Saglikli Yasa*'s success came from the personal networks within the group and the key role they played in facilitating the group's involvement in policy-making. The work *Saglikli Yasa* undertook with regard to social affairs was facilitated by informal links with welfare organizations and the senate. It was these personal linkages, paired with a migrant-friendly attitude in the bureau of public health, which facilitated the larger groups' access to policy forums and helped to provide access to government funding.

The second group's involvement in health care policy-making started with its engagement in informal government dialogues that resulted in the granting of state funding for migrant-specific mental health care structures. Formed in the 1980s, the *Institut für Psychosoziale Arbeit und Prävention* (IPAP or Institute for

7 Organized by Meyer and the bureau of public health.

8 This center later became Refugio—a nation-wide NGO that is financed by regional and EU funding.

Psychosocial Work and Prevention) became the first institution in Bremen that offered multilingual mental health care services for citizens with a background of migration. IPAP employed Turkish- and Arabic-speaking psychologists from the *Saglikli Yasa* circle, and in 1992 organized a conference on migration and psychosocial health. The IPAP group, whose main title became DEVA, an Arabic/Turkish word that translates as "path toward solution" or "cure," is the only group that indirectly and directly contributed to the establishment of state-funded migrant-specific health services in Bremen. The third group that was involved in policy-making in the widest sense forwarded their concerns about establishing a mental health center for immigrants to the government. At first, the government showed great interest in the center; however, it never supported the implementation of this project. Despite the fact that the bureau acknowledged that immigrants faced higher access barriers than non-immigrants, a lack of political will and a shortage of financial resources prevented action on the proposed center. Instead, the bureau of public health recommended the establishment of a public discussion forum on migrants and mental health. The overall neglect of migrant-specific care in Bremen is based on a universalist discursive frame in which the availability of access is declared to be equally available to all citizens. In line with this discourse, the government terminated DEVA's[9] funding in 2006, putting an end to the only migrant-organized and non-refugee focused migrant-specific health service in Bremen.

In 2005, when migration rates to Bremen had further increased, two migrant-specific services (psychological counseling in Russian and Turkish) were established in Bremen hospitals as a response to migrant-related pressure on the health care system. This happened as a result of the initiative taken by two medical directors confronted with a high number of patients with a background of migration—many of whom have poor German language skills and therefore face difficulties in treatment. One of the reasons why the creation of migrant-friendly structures was suddenly possible was the directors' awareness of migrant's needs, paired with their structural positioning within the hospital and within the city-state. This positioning gave them access to informal meetings with government representatives. Specifically, good relations with the bureau of public health (one of the main funding institutions for such services by then) played a facilitating role, as confirmed to us by one of the bureau's leading figures.

However, further events influenced the Bremen health care system toward accommodating the concerns of migrants more fully. In 2007, a two-day conference on migration and health was organized by a research group on migration and health at the University of Bremen in cooperation with the EU-funded XENOS group: *Leben und Arbeiten in Vielfalt: Gesundheit Interkulturelle* (Living and Working in Diversity: Health Intercultural). The conference, which addressed the issue of intercultural competence in the health care system and aimed to create

9 IPAB was renamed and is now called DEVA. For matters of clarity, we refer to it as IPAB throughout the chapter.

awareness about immigrants' access barriers to hospitals, targeted hospital staff, health experts and policy-makers. Central results from the conference were its participants' claims to establish migrant-friendly health care structures in Bremen. The requests concerned the provision of translation services, affirmative action, diversity training and generally the creation of space and tolerance for religious and cultural diversity. Conference participants also articulated the need to work more closely with migrant communities and to create an all-embracing network of health providers among those who deal with migrants in Bremen.

A year later, in March 2008, the working group that had emerged from the conference, together with other migration and health-related institutions, founded the Interkulturelles Gesundheitsnetzwerk Bremen (Intercultural Health Network of Bremen). Members of the network are health care institutions from the public sector, as well as experts, decision-makers and migrant representatives who work with migrants and are aware of their health care access barriers. The network is divided into ten new working groups which regularly convene with the overall aim of creating equality of chances and improving the health-related and psychosocial situation of migrants living in Bremen. Until 2011 the network was coordinated by a member of the bureau of public health and is approved by the state, but receives no government funding. Emerging from the network are planning sessions for round table talks with hospital directors. These talks were planned by the network, in cooperation with the senate and the hospital society with the aim to improve migrants' access to health care by inserting migrant-friendliness into the quality assurance system of Bremen's hospitals. In the end however they were cancelled for lack of interest from the side of the hospitals and the senate who argued that hospitals are already sufficiently migrant-friendly. This initiative nevertheless demonstrates the role of grassroots groups that, to a large degree from within the health care system, organize to bring about incremental institutional change in response to the challenge of cultural diversity.

The situation of migrants in Leipzig today is comparable to that of migrants in Bremen in the 1970s. The majority of migrant organizations still operate on a local level that is characterized by loosely organized, grassroots citizen groups with no contact to government policy-making. Regular health-related self-help groups do not exist at the city level and health-related services operate within the framework of informal support networks. Cultural requests are highlighted in the field of maternal care and mental health. Especially in the psychotherapy sector, pro-migrant groups articulate requests that advocate a more migrant-specific health supply. In our interviews, health experts mentioned that patients from the Near and Middle East face particularly great access barriers due to cultural taboos. Only one of the hospitals offers psychiatric services (Verbund gemeindenaher Psychiatrie) for female ethnic Germans, an offer initiated by an employee with a migration background. And though many migrants show a preference for doctors from their country of origin, the organizations do not address these requests. Rather, they promote the integration of migrant-specific health structures into the regular services.

The claims of the Vietnamese community address equal access to medical universities, due to a 0 percent ratio of Vietnamese medical doctors to the Vietnamese migrant community (which constitutes the largest in Leipzig). Migrant organizations that work on a regional level with a broader network of contacts claim political participation. The RAA (Regional Office for Questions of Foreigners and Ethnic German Migrants/ SALVE) association, for instance, promotes the establishment of a council for migration. Though unsuccessfully, the Association of Foreign Citizens claimed funding for extra health insurance advances from the labor office. Hence, even in Leipzig migrants have entered into a dialogue with health care decision-makers and the policy community, though with less tangible outcomes. They nevertheless contributed to the lowering of access barriers for migrants by establishing short-term migrant-specific services, such as translation services in medical institutions.

Like in Bremen, leftist pro-migrant organizations in Leipzig are also involved in political claim-making, as well as in service delivery. For instance, they focus on improving asylum seekers' food provision. The "*Umtauschinitiative*," a grassroots pro-migrant association, initiated the replacement of food vouchers with cash to facilitate free food choice for asylum seekers. The focus of these organizations from the leftist spectrum of civil society is predominantly targeted at providing marginalized migrant groups (most notably refugees and irregular migrants) with adequate and accessible health care services. Again, it is the universalist discursive framework (with its emphasis on inclusiveness and fairness), rather than the idea of group-specific rights or services, that drives the agenda.

Unlike in Bremen, where migrants had already organized practitioners' conferences in the 1980s, the first comparable workshop in Leipzig only took place in 2006. Organized by the department of Medical Psychology and Medical Sociology at the University of Leipzig, it constituted the first exchange forum for scientists, politicians and practitioners working on the issue of migration and health in Leipzig. During this workshop, medical directors, representatives of migrant organizations, pro-migrant organizations from Leipzig and experts on migrant health research from other cities discussed migrants' health needs and barriers in the city. A focus of the workshop was on asylum-seekers and refugees. However, while the conference helped to raise awareness on the topic, no political claims emerged from it and structural changes were only indirectly implemented.[10]

Political Advocacy

By trying to analyze migrants' level of participation in Bremen, we have seen that they started to organize their interests, raise awareness and offer migrant-specific services through their organizations alongside and complementing the health care system. When it comes to structural changes through formal participatory

10 Members of the study group established a temporary translators pool for health services that was active from 2006–2008.

procedures on higher levels (such as the establishment of migrant-specific services in hospitals), however, their area of influence remains limited. Here, individual Germans and their established network in the political arena of Bremen turned out to be the central factor for change. When it comes to the foundation of the intercultural health network and the organization of round table talks, a multitude of issues contributed to change. The ongoing paradigm change within the German health care system was an important asset that affected the changing attitude toward migrants on the regional level in terms of the recognition of migrants needs. Besides the environment conducive for change this created, the continuous increase in national and global interest in the issue of migration created a greater availability of research funding.

It is in this context that we have to understand the empowerment of civil society groups (such as XENOS) through funding as a major motor mobilizing civil engagement for the issue. In many ways the issue encountered fertile grounds and due to the availability of funding, was made subject to facilitate participatory forums. A comparative advantage was also a certain neutrality of these actors as bodies that, unlike most other actors, did not compete over government funding and were not part of a network of alliances. All of the above-mentioned factors contributed to the establishment of the intercultural health network in Bremen as the first public forum that managed to bring together a considerably large group of diverse actors on the issue.

Migrants' organizations role in this process was to help create awareness and to lower access barriers for migrants by establishing services. Importantly, they initiated the emergence of a discursive frame and hence awareness about immigrants' needs at the city level, which corresponded and interacted with a changing awareness about the need for migrant-friendly health care on the national level. It is in this sense that migrants, along with other pro-migrant groups, indirectly contributed to the structural changes enacted by the two German assistant medical directors in Bremen. Along with non-migrants, they started participating in the policy-making process in the sense that important state-and non-state actors are now actively involved in improving migrants' access to health care.

Though decision-makers in Leipzig hardly contributed to infrastructural changes in Leipzig, our interviews strongly suggest that the perception of migrants in the city has changed. Though structural changes have not taken place, migration as an issue of public interest has entered the public sphere in form of events, activities and representations. One of the few positive examples of concrete responsiveness toward migrants' needs was the establishment of mother language-based school programs for Vietnamese migrants in Leipzig (for a more detailed description of a positive example, see Chapter 5).[11]

11 In sharp contrast stand the unsuccessful funding requests of the head of the Association for Foreign Citizens. Apart from the response of a regional bank and a political party respectively offering 150 Euros, neither companies nor political parties reacted to this request, indicating the low level of interest in supporting migrant issues.

Compared to the non-migrant friendly political landscape, we find that claim-making results of migrants and pro-migrant groups are rather tokenistic in Saxon cities. While the necessity of addressing the issue of cultural diversity in the health care system was underlined by many of our interviewees, institutional reforms and new services are still very limited in scope.

While state authorities often proved unresponsive to the claims of migrant organizations, the latter proved to be widely dependent on state subsidies. Indeed, a high level of competition over resources has partly paralyzed joint efforts and participation in policy-making and the establishment of network structures in Bremen.[12] Involvement in the policy-making process is highly influenced by alliances between individual actors within the government departments. Rather than organized interests, it is often these personalized links which play a significant role in channeling resources and orienting policy-makers' funding decisions. When it comes to the direct political participation of migrants in policy-making processes, we observe a lack of encouragement by the state.

Although informal networks and contacts with political decision-makers partly exist in Leipzig, the cooperation usually suffers from the lack of formalized relationships between migrant associations and city representatives. In addition, difficulties in exerting policy-shaping influence are compounded by the fact that migrant organizations in Leipzig keep only limited links with the national level and do not cooperate with government organizations.

To summarize the main points illustrated by the German case and as already alluded to at a more general level in the previous chapter, there is a notable gap between the national discourse on culturally-sensitive integration and political participation on the one hand, and how these principles are implemented on the ground in particular urban contexts on the other. There is simply no homogeneous national model structuring the engagement of migrants and their organizations within the health care system. Rather, what we found in our two case studies is a wide variety in terms of modes of engagement, the types of actors involved and the responses from policy authorities. Many of the initiatives for implementing change in the health care sector come from small groups (often represented by highly-motivated health care professionals or civil society activists) that take advantage of opportunities for change that are more specific to the local context and less a structural opening within mainstream institutions of policy processes. Still, all dimensions of migrants' engagement (information provision, advocacy and service delivery) are present, even if they are performed with different levels of efficiency and centrality. Advocacy capabilities in particular are limited. One important variable is the greater prominence of older migrant associations with substantial social capital and societal incorporation of the relevant ethnic groups, such as Turkish associations.

12 The city of Bremen is one of the most indebted German cities and faces severe financial shortages. Besides, competition over resources is high due to Bremen's small size and its status as a city state.

Participation in Health Care: The Case of Italy

Current policy approaches to migrants' health have their roots in the events of the early 1990s. In those years, the first large wave of migrants that had arrived in the 1980s was gradually becoming stably incorporated into workplaces and social institutions, and the issue of their access to health provisions was being tackled. Decision-making processes of the early 1990s were influenced by the activism of volunteers and associations that played an important role in guaranteeing the health care of migrants, regular and irregular, and were crucial for the creation of more inclusive norms. Only later would this process of awareness-raising involve public actors. When private social and volunteer organizations operating at the local level increased their ability to cooperate, spread information and put pressure on institutions during the 1990s, they also managed to push from the bottom in the field of health care. Their aim was to improve access for legal and irregular migrants, reorganizing health and social services and reorienting it to identify the risk factors for foreigners coming to Italy. During our analysis, the weak role played by migrants in health policy-making also clearly emerged. It is of particular importance to note the absence of these associations in the initial policy-shaping stage.

In this period and also later, the main civil society actor was the *Società Italiana di Medicina delle Migrazioni* (*SIMM* or Italian Society for Migrants' Medicine), which was founded in 1990 by a small group of doctors and voluntary operators (none of them with a background of migration), who, in different Italian cities, supported migrant patients and sought to raise social awareness of issues related to their health. The society has the aim of: promoting, linking and coordinating health activities for migrants; encouraging study and research in the field of migrants' medicine; starting a "forum" for the sharing, at national and international levels, of information and methodologies of approach to migrant patients; and sponsoring training activities in the field of health protection of migrants' health (from the Statute of SIMM).

Thanks to its activities during the 1990s, SIMM built an association network gathering hundreds of people (experts in various fields and representatives of important agencies at the national level), improving coordination and information exchange between all the associations spread across the national territory. In contrast to other policy sectors, it must be highlighted that associations committed to the health care field were able to unite under one subject: forming a compact network able to organize lobbying activities aimed at institutions. Though there are different views about some topics and approaches between the different subjects both inside SIMM and between SIMM and other associations in the field, they were able to jointly confront institutions and elaborate shared proposals, often finding a positive response.

Although there was no institutional access to the decision-making process, in the early 1990s the network of contacts built by the associations provided the path toward productive cooperation with Health Minister Guzzanti (1994–1996). The involvement of some MPs and of the Minister moved the Senate to charge the Dini government to "search forms of defending the right to health for non-EU citizens, by issuing acts able to overcome the obstacles that in practice prevent the equality of treatments" (Geraci 2005: 61). Therefore, the turning point in the health care policy for migrants started in 1995: Thanks to SIMM's personal relations, Minister of Health Guzzanti, in cooperation with Caritas of Rome, welcomed the proposal of the associations and introduced a norm establishing that a foreigner present in Italy is entitled to health care, even without a residence permit and without risking being reported to the police after the treatment (Chapter 4).[13] Later, during the center-left government, the associations found institutional access channels and several representatives could participate in the preparing workshops for the Turco-Napolitano law (1998) and other consultative commissions. These opportunities established the concept of "health citizenship"—conceptualizing health as a fundamental aspect of social rights. Associations emphasized the importance of health rights. Therefore, health provisions were written on the basis of the results of the preparatory meetings with the representatives of some volunteers' associations working in the field. The following was the opinion of a physician (a member of SIMM and then-consultant for the Health Ministry) who participated in the writing of the articles of the Turco-Napolitano law that pertain to health care:

> … a pressure at national level, because in those years we asked to dialogue with the Health Ministry, we were heard and we exposed our viewpoints, I highlighted the question, strategically effective, of clandestine people. The argument of public health care, which underlines how the care of the community means caring about everyone, whoever she/he is, whatever is her/his entitlement, and for whatever reason she/he is present in the country was an argument that the Minister of the time could support even politically, because he was influential and had scientific credibility also towards the political parties who mostly opposed to open toward irregular immigrants, and this was very important. (Physician, Rome, 2006)

Another crucial actor in the debate between the associations and the ministry was the President of SIMM, who was responsible for the health sector of Caritas and also underlined that:

---

13 Article 13 of the Decree says: "Foreigners temporarily present in the territory of the State are entitled to continuous health care in the public health services, surgery and hospital care in case of illness or accidents and all the preventative medicine programs. The social protection of maternity and pregnancy is also guaranteed … The access to the health structures for foreigners cannot involve any type of reporting, except when a medical report is compulsory, with equal conditions as those requested for Italian citizens. Except for the participatory fees, if required, the preventative treatments, the maternity and pregnancy, care and all the other treatments mentioned by the health minister decree, are all free of charge for the applicant … within the national health funding, by using if necessary, part of the resources destined to the health emergency and within the limits of health care levels."

> [I]t was a real battle about that … It was a period I remember being in meetings lasting until four at night, and fights and fights and fights … Some of the results of this battle you can see in the law, because there are some passages that you can't understand; very ambiguous, because they came out of compromises and of interpretations. (Caritas Rome, 2006)

Although juridical tools were sufficiently developed, at the end of the 1990s the implementation of legislative dispositions was still not everywhere guaranteed at the local level. In every area the situation depended on a different combination of practices, resources, sensibility and training. Trying to give more homogeneity to the organization of services, in 1998 Minister of Health Bindi promoted and encouraged the creation of a "discussion table." This consultative forum was formed by regional representatives with the important task of managing the connection among the national and regional level of the Italian National Health System, and, within the National Coordination Body (ONC), of a working group of experts named "*Gruppo di Lavoro Salute e Immigrazione*" (Working Group on Labour, Health and Immigration) which handled the tasks of comparing the normative and statistical data on migrants and discussing future projects. The Group, analyzing some specific local areas and taking into account the needs of local institutions' administrators and managers of health units, concentrated on the theme of access to health services. They elaborated proposals and set out priorities for the local level, such as: training of personnel; interpretation of needs and demands; organization of services; flexibility of the offer; multidisciplinary work; and network operations. This team worked on the preparation of the health plan for the years 1998–2000 (where migrants were included for the first time among the weak subjects for specific actions) and committed itself to the preparation of two reports on immigrants' health conditions. Using all of the available data on the health conditions of migrants, a survey on their hospitalization (with disaggregated data on foreigners) was conducted for the first time.

However, this initially encouraging situation soon faced some challenges, as, both in the Group "Health and Immigration" and in the consultations of the Ministry, not all expectations and requests of associations were fulfilled. According to SIMM's President and one representative of the *Istituto Superiore di Sanità* (High Institute of Health), the limits were implicit in the highly bureaucratic approach of administrators and officers who often showed little interest in the topic:

> Those who deal with these questions are often people, like ministries' officers, who have no idea of what there is outside. They are excellent in codes, codicils, laws, etcetera, and so they can arrange very, very consistent stuff, but they don't have any perception of what the real problem is. (Caritas Rome, May, 2006)

> Sometimes we are called to meet in consultative meetings, but this doesn't mean that what comes out is going to be actually used. Sometimes yes, but it seems to me that it's a question of being lucky, with mysterious mechanisms

> that I can't always understand. Sometimes everything goes smoothly. Often we publish very good documents, such as the project maternal-child-objective, a document existing since 1998, written in 1998 and come out in 2000, where there are excellent suggestions … But then passing from what is written to its implementation … a lot of time passes or it's not made, in brief, many things remain in name only. (Researcher of Health Superior Institute, Rome, May 2006)

The legislative interventions of the center-right government (for example, with Act 189 of July 30, 2002 also called the "Bossi-Fini" Law) did not modify the norms on migrants' health care. However, although the norms on health care are generally considered to be excellent, they are to be considered in the normative background on immigration, which is now stricter due to the changes introduced by the center-right government. According to many experts, these changes contribute to making migrants' social life more fragile and therefore, indirectly, to worsening their health conditions. According to the interviewees, the inactivity of the commissions charged with consulting immigrants' representatives after 2001 further weakened their participation:

> Their (immigrant) associations are not very effective. They aren't very active in this field and unfortunately in the last five years, with the government we had, the commissions where they were present were cancelled. For example, there was a commission of the Council of Ministers and another of the Ministry of Health—those were excellent occasions and there were some immigrants. But in the five years of Berlusconi government nothing more was made. These commissions, though foreseen by the law, were never summoned up. (Physician, Migrant Association, Trento, 2006)

Besides, over the last few years corresponding to the legislature guided by the center-right (2001–2006), the dialogue and participation opportunities were greatly reduced in the field of health care as well. The main consultative structures were a Commission for the Integration of Immigrants and a Consultative Committee for Immigrants (Zincone 2001). Both were terminated. The National Coordination Body and the roundtable formed by regional representatives were rarely summoned up and functioned intermittently, though our informants considered them the best place for sharing best practices and problems. The closure of the channels of dialogue at the national level during the center-right government was the main concern of the majority of the associations' representatives that we interviewed. The feeling among those interviewed was that the reasons for this discontinuation of both the Commission for the Integration of Immigrants and the Consultative Committee for Immigrants were political and that decision-makers were willfully seeking to renounce responsibility for integrating immigrants and combating discrimination. They felt that this was a calculated political choice on the part of decision-makers to gain electoral advantage. The principal criticisms regarding the political system among those interviewed were: the lack of interest in dialogue; the increased weight given to the financing of security and control measures regarding immigrants, while at the same time funds for integration purposes were decreased. As an ethno-psychiatrist and member of SIMM's managing board declared:

> [W]e strongly lobbied at different levels, on central and regional governments, obviously with changing results according to the government, when center-left we got a lot, when center-right zero, but really zero at central level, while we got much from regional governments ... we get on better with center-left regional ones but that's not always guaranteed. (Physician, Migrant Association, Trento, 2006)

With the first commitments of the new center-left government (2006–2008), the pro-migrant associations hoped to regain influence, but the rise of a new center-right government after 2008 further limited their impact.

Due to difficulties in dialogue at the national level and waiting for the start of a coordinating table among the regions which began in 1998, SIMM has in recent years reinforced its lobbying activities at the local level, promoting the connections between different groups working in the field for the protection of foreigners' health. The policy-shaping tool promoted by SIMM was the creation of local groups, called *Gruppi Regionali Immigrazione e Salute* (*GRIS* or "Regional Groups on Immigration and Health"). These are grassroots groups of Italians and non-Italians working for the promotion of migrants' health care. Such groups work with the aim of making health services accessible and usable for all. To be effective, the existence of the right of access must be accompanied by the consciousness of being entitled to the right itself and by the possibility of enforcing it. The immigrant, therefore, must be informed and orientated toward services, and actions to overcome barriers in access to health care must be implemented. Such groups were activated in various regions (Lazio, Sardinia, Sicily, Lombardy and Veneto) and in the Provinces of Trento and Bolzano, but similar networks, more or less structured, are also present in other local areas: "The function of GRIS is to reach policies shared by institutions and different worlds, such as associations and immigrants' groups reclaiming and expecting some of the rights that are not yet perceived as such" (ISMU Manager, Professor at the Faculty of Political Sciences of Milan, 2006).

In the years following the 2008 election of a new center-right government, the situation has evolved, although not significantly in legislative terms. The new government has from the beginning appeared more concerned with stopping immigration—particularly irregular immigration—than with improving access to health and other services, which at least a part of the government coalition saw as so exceedingly generous that it encouraged irregular migration. In terms of political culture, the new ruling coalition has been characterized by the principles of the Bossi-Fini law (n. 189/2002), which emphasizes a conceptualization of the migrant as a worker and connects migrants' entitlements to this social function, rather than to a broader vision of social citizenship. The coalition also sees migrants primarily as a threat to security. A policy initiative along these lines, called the "security package," passed a 2009 vote and modified aspects of the legislation on immigration. It introduced the concept of irregular immigration as a punishable crime. It imposed new obstacles to the acquisition of Italian citizenship, such as under certain conditions the obligation to demonstrate knowledge of the Italian language. It legitimated private vigilante groups, which have often been publicly perceived as aimed at migrants' crime. Notably, in the field of health it sought to abolish the prohibition on reporting to the police irregular migrants who seek medical assistance. However, this attempt activated a widespread mobilization which involved professional health bodies, universities, civil society groups and center and center-left political parties. Ten regional councils expressed their unwillingness to comply with the new dispositions. As a consequence of this extensive mobilization, in April 2009 this disposition was eliminated from the "security package." However, this elimination created substantial normative ambiguity. As irregular immigration is now a crime, public officials are formally obliged to report irregular migrants. However, because of the absence of a specific disposition, this norm might not be applicable to the field of health. In this context of legislative uncertainty, public authorities have been acting inconsistently across different regions. Until 2010, 14 regional councils have expressed the formal view that the prohibition on reporting irregular migrants accessing health services remains. However, to the extent that other regions have not done so, substantial uncertainty remains and thus limits migrants' willingness to seek medical assistance.[14]

The broader situation of migrants' engagement in Italy over the two decades can be described both in terms of normalization and polarization. First, from the onset of migration flows since the early 1990s, their role in public and political life has gradually expanded and become a normalized feature in civil society. One can identify typical patterns of exchanges between civil society and the political system in terms of informational exchanges, patterns of deployment of influence and service associated, albeit with a limited degree of migrants' empowerment. In Italy, advocacy on behalf of migrants proves to be strongly connected to traditional actors in society that are routinely associated with the left. Second, the current situation can best be described as one of polarization between a supportive political and organizational environment for migrants and their associations on the one hand, and a popular public opinion and dominant section of the political environment that is much less favorable on the other.

Functions and Limits of Italian Civil Society in Health Care

Engagement: The limited interaction with the policy community

As in other migration-related fields, in the field of health policy a productive informational exchange between civil society and decision-making institutions

14 See Geraci et al. (2010).

is limited by the small size and overall limited relevance of consultative fora (*Fondazione Corazzin* 2001).

In addition, there are intractable difficulties with regard to the identification of representatives. The nomination of foreign representatives for health-related consultative commissions at a national level (in the years when those bodies were active) did not systematically involve immigrant communities or associations. These representatives were chosen not through representative elections, but through co-optation by ministries which chose their interlocutors on the basis of their expertise (such as physicians or professionals working in hospitals) or, more simply, on the basis of personal relationships built over time (in other commissions or during public meetings or debates).

To the question about the participation level of immigrants in consultative and decisional bodies, the unanimous answer was that they are not sufficiently represented. For example, a teacher who is an expert in the field declared:

> I still don't see them as well integrated. I still see them in a situation of exclusion. Also, from the social point of view and from the cultural point of view, they seem to me somehow still very ghettoized, so their claims are today still very elementary … We are still in a situation of first generation and of big fragmentation of policies … I find that they don't have yet the status of a pressure or interest group able to influence national, local or territorial policies (ISMU Manager, Professor at the Faculty of Political Sciences of Milan, 2006)

This description reflects a recurrent pattern that we found in all of the contexts investigated. The interviewed representatives of pro-migrants' associations declared that whenever they tried to interact with immigrant communities in order to encourage their participation, they discovered migrants had a great lack of knowledge about their own rights. The most necessary activity for migrants' communities (and also for irregular migrants) still seems to be the diffusion of information about rights guaranteeing their access to health services, preventative programs (screening, smear-test, inoculations) and programs to prepare for childbirth. Moreover, the interviewees underlined the necessity of increasing the associations' competences in dealing with public institutions and services and encouraging participation in public life:

> As I wrote in the reports of the Commission for Integration, the perspective was to consolidate channels of exchange, communication, cooperation with all the communities at all possible levels. Of course this is not easy, because first of all there is the discourse of empowerment of the existing communities, and then there is the question of identifying the most practical forms of cooperation. (Consultant for the Ministry, Agenzia di Sanità Pubblica della Regione Lazio, Rome, 2006)

Other interviewees affirm instead that the topic of health care is not considered crucial by immigrants because, notwithstanding the problems of communication, access and usability, health assistance is generally guaranteed to everyone. This is, for example, the opinion of a researcher of the Health Superior Institute:

> I think they don't express themselves about health because on one hand they are a young and healthy population, so it is much more urgent for them to find a house, some food, a job, or a permit of stay than going to a physician, even though they have some tooth-ache. Also because they are generally quite healthy and if in the end they go to our first aid services … must wait for five hours, they nevertheless got something and also for free. If they go to free gynecological clinics ('consultori') they'll have to wait for some days but they manage to be visited. They go to [the] hospital for giving birth and they're very happy because they say 'I wish it was like this in our country'. (Researcher of Health Superior Institute, Rome, 2006)

At the local level, the main supporters of migrants' interests, acting as bridges for the requests made by ethnic associations, are still associations and cooperatives settled by Italians. Thus, the knowledge that policy-makers can acquire from civil society organizations is limited in the case of migrant interlocutors by the fact that they are not necessarily representative of their communities, and in the case of associational interlocutors by the fact that they might not know what are the issues most relevant to specific ethnic communities. However, several interviewees point out that no viable solution to the problem of representativeness is available in the absence of community cohesion. Several interviewees argue that in the present context, a representation of migrant communities that is in any way mediated by existing migrant associations is not going to produce a real representation of the issues and views of ethnic groups. Rather, it is going to ensure that the representation of migrants remains formal rather than substantial:

> That is another flaw of local level policies. First we should ask them: 'Excuse us, what do you need?' We always have the Eurocentric perspective flaw of thinking in the name of, and on behalf of … that is, it's us who prepare the services for migrants, without listening to them. And even the existing consultative bodies, such as the Regional Consultation Organization (Consulta) for immigration, become meaningless. This is because they do not participate in a real consultation process. They are not really consulted on interventions to be made … Yes, there are foreign trade unionists, but the trade unionists are merely there to represent the union. In fact, too often I complained that there are no migrants in this permanent Council … If we analyze the Ivory Coast, we see that they are all divided in so many groups. The same applies to the Senegalese, the Tamil, the Sri Lankan; there are differences. What I mean is that often the representative of migrants ends up only representing himself. But if we go into

> the communities and ask: 'Is that your representative?' they would say: 'who knows him?' (Activist, Migrant Association, Naples, 2006)

> The more migrants are represented, the more their problems are realistically presented because there is no one better to talk about problems than those who live through them and talk about their need and the adequate institutional responses they receive. When we talk about migrants we put them all in the same box, but migrants are not all the same. Problems faced by women are different from those of men and children, also because of their different origins and lifestyles. Not all migrants share the same problems and face them in the same way. For example, accessing services is not the same for a Moldovan or a Moroccan woman because they have different ideas on how to face a pregnancy. Therefore, when we talk about migrants we have to pay attention to who we are talking about. Therefore, the more associations [that] are represented within GRIS, the more problems can be addressed. There is the equality of rights, everyone has the right to access health care, but not everyone has the same needs or not everyone accesses them in the same way. (Activist, Migrant Association, Naples, 2006)

However, significant differences were evident in different territorial contexts. Immigrants who settled in Trento experienced a local political system particularly capable of both stimulating forms of institutional representation and facilitating a transition from informal to formal networks among associations. The system generally supports effective participation practices and provides more chances to participate in the policy process. In the case of Trento, in fact, a prominent role is played by GRIS. Here, the immigrant communities that came earlier and are better settled in the area show more interest by proposing clear issues and cultural and ethnic requests, as evidenced by the Islamic Community and multi-ethnic associations of health mediation (often composed by women) cooperating with the local health unit. In the case of Naples, where the network is less structured and the role of public institutions is more central, a prominent role is played by single migrants who work as mediators in Italian or mixed cooperatives, or in the trade unions. In both cities, a relevant (but still unsung) role is also played by physicians with a background of migration, who are already Italian citizens and work for the national health service (Servizio Sanitario Nazionale-SSN) and who, over the years, took on an active role in mixed associations. Nonetheless, even in Trento migrants' associational participation in health policy remains limited.

According to some interviewees, the lack of participation of migrants' associations can be explained mainly in terms of more important needs to be satisfied in other fields (education, employment, housing) and as more essential for the integration process. In the Italian context migrants tend to view health problems only when their health is already compromised, dealing with single cases inside the community rather than as a general issue.

Advocacy and Political Awareness

One of the most interesting aspects that emerged during our analysis is the different forms of participation offered by institutions to pro-migrant associations since the 1990s. During the center-left governments (1996–2001; 2006–2008), participation was widened by the creation of advisory committees and bodies including many people, and opened to whoever was interested. In the years of center-left government, we witnessed a greater involvement of associations at the institutional level. Institutions appeared to be willing to include civil society associations mainly because they were dependent on them for expertise and information on specific issues. The need for information, in particular, seems to be the decisive factor shaping the behavior of public decision-making bodies (Marks 1996: 61). Thanks to their expertise on the subject, pressure groups do have a great advantage to government bodies that need essential help with their administrative and legislative activities. In a context of vague and uncertain political processes, the experts' values become especially influential and, if their ideas are shared by political decision-makers, their efficacy is greater (Majone 1989; Ruzza 2005). In the case we examined, the influence of SIMM's physicians was particularly strong.

During the center-right government of 2001–2006, consulting and community outreach was promoted less and included fewer people; consultants were mainly chosen on the basis of their technical experience. Broader consultation increased during the center-left years and decreased again after the center-right success in 2008. What clearly emerged in all cases is a tension between representativeness and efficiency—these can be conceptualized as two distinctive forms of participation. Participants can be the few available technically-trained professionals, or they can be wider civil society representatives who abound in numbers but often lack specific competences. Representation, if widened too much, produces difficulties in coordinating the different subjects involved, while technical competence criterion, if too narrow, reduces the possibility of expressing the full range of societal views. This contrast can be mapped to political orientation. In this sense, SIMM's President highlighted that consulting activities encountered a series of limits, both with center-left and center-right governments:

> [W]ith center-left there is a hyper-participation, becoming nearly confusion. With center-right there is a focused participation, aimed at only one thing and only with chosen people. And this was a problem for us, sometimes, because we are for a widened participation but widened to people somehow competent … When you have to talk about technical aspects, assemblies are not useful. (Caritas Rome, May 2006)

It should be pointed out that the technical skills of participants in high-level consultations with the government on migration policy proved essential in several cases. For instance, during the center-left government, SIMM strived to provide relevant information and exerted advocacy to persuade political actors inclined to desist from taking a hard line on the planned expulsion of migrants:

> [A]t that time they wanted to expel a woman as soon as her baby was three months old. Then I said: 'I am a doctor, I don't know if there are other colleagues in this commission, but I don't know if you realize what is a three months' baby, what are the cares he needs and what can mean an expulsion for a mother with such a young baby.' And so we fought for widening this disposal. Then we obtained just a half, but we managed to further procrastinate the expulsion scheduling. (Consultant for the Ministry, Agenzia di Sanità Pubblica della Regione Lazio, Rome, 2006)

On this topic, a physician and member of SIMM's managing board underlined the importance of the strong credibility of his association, a credibility which often enabled him to obtain policy results without engaging in conflict with political actors:

> I don't think that the approaches are so different; we are all for the rights and for health care. The question is rather the procedures to be followed. Perhaps we have the advantage of a credibility built along 16 years … and also another advantage, in my opinion, is that we are quite good in dealing with politicians … [W]ith them you must not be too demanding, you have to be able to reason in political terms … and to make compromises. Turco-Napolitano law is a law which left enormous voids, which didn't grant citizenship nor vote. There isn't a law about asylum; in other words there are very serious lacks, but at that time we could have taken very firm positions and say 'No!' … It's important to be open to compromise, to mediate, to debate, to accept compromises, so we didn't manage to obtain these things. But we obtained a health legislation that, I think, is the most advanced in Europe, maybe in the world, I don't know … So it's fundamental to have the capacity of negotiating, of being diplomatic, of accepting compromise. Sometimes some colleagues, even very generous ones, clash openly with these situations and they remain empty handed, because they provoke a rigid reaction in the political counterpart, so … we had to reach a compromise. (Physician, Migrant Association, Milan, 2006)[15]

By contrast, other associations active in the field of health care or dealing more generally with immigration, exercise more antagonistic forms of pressure (a range of confrontational and non-confrontational tactics are utilized):

---

15 Mr Storace is a well-known right-wing politician who used to be an MP in the center-right party Alleanza Nazionale (AN) and in 2007 funded a new right-wing party called "La Destra" (The Right).

> When we have common goals we often get in conflict about the methodologies to reach them, about how to deal with some aspects. We get on quite well with trade unions even if we criticize them a lot, because anyway they don't do enough: On one hand, immigrants are everyday more and more inside trade unions. On the other hand, there is a lack of safeguarding the weak categories. With the Catholic Church we have a dialogue; in lots of areas priests are the only representatives of a civic society often in the front line. But there is a basic difference because they anyway try to create charity systems and we don't agree on that. We are for the promotion of a right. (Representative of Doctors Without Borders/Médecins Sans Frontières, April 2006)

Our interviews showed that in local contexts, *advocacy* activities are carried out by established networks whenever these are available. For example, in Trento advocacy is delegated to GRIS. Migrants' associations prefer to use GRIS because this organization gathers the views of various associations and therefore has more representative power, and also because it has more experience in mediation and negotiation with political institutions. Other migrants' associations are still weak, as migrants are at the initial phase of social integration:

> We come from countries where there are few or no associations; therefore, we wanted someone to help us along the way … Thus, as a group we did exist even a year before, but we waited until we found someone who helped us and showed the way, the potentiality for consultancies, the way to draw statuses and other things. We were lacking expertise. (AMIC)

Contacts with the health authority by representatives of migrants' associations are just beginning. At this stage they are mainly used at the level of *informants* in order to understand organizational needs and to obtain suggestions to improve the access to the health services, without any space for "groups" (either ethnic or not) in the decision-making process.

> I think that our task is also that (thanks to the contacts and interaction with these associations and representatives of migrants) of knowing the reality, knowing how to act in order to facilitate. Our main goal is knowledge. We are a complex system that deals with various carriers of specific interests. All these carriers, in various forms, have to be listened to and then when decisions are made they should include their opinions, even though obviously in the end we will make the decisions. Therefore, in dealing with these migrants' associations, we behave in the same way as we would with Italian associations, for example those of diabetics or of hospital care …
>
> It's obvious that if there is an association with its beautiful statute, we ask for it and then this association is entered in our database of associations and when we consult the organizations, we invite them too. Thus, we cannot have

> relationships with four hundred eighty thousand citizens—it's obvious—but if someone says something, or goes to the 'office of contacts with the public' and talks to … if he/she says sensible things we take them into account. (Political administrator, Trento, 2005)

As far as activities of *policy-making are concerned*, the role of migrants' associations in Naples is very limited. On the few occasions when it took place, it was mainly for consultations during meetings where the main interest of institutions was to assemble the biggest number of migrants (in order to justify the interventions), rather than to effectively listen to their opinions.

Therefore, the institutions and mechanisms put in place seem to be interested more in doing something "for" the migrants than "with" the migrants. Some associations are also registered with the Regional Consultation for Immigration and the Local Territorial Council in Naples, but, according to the interviewees, they stay at the margin in the definition of migrants' policies. This is how a representative of a migrants' association and a migrant trade unionist express it:

> … [The councilor] calls you when there are meetings and needs to have numbers and to be able to say that migrants' associations are present, and possibly say that migrants did not fully understand. Councilors made us create the associations, gave us a lot to of trouble to keep them, forced us make final reports, attend the meetings and today the existence of the association does not take us anywhere because it is the Council that makes every decision.

> The migrants' associations are not very active in politics—they dedicate themselves to other activities, such as cuisine, music, or anything, don't they? Furthermore, at the local council there are only few associations represented—only two—and this creates conflicts with the territorial council, which never meets anyway. The last time it met was a long time ago. Even when we signed an agreement on health that was very important, the associations involved were only two. Then there were the unions, the local council, a range of organizations which are more institutionalized, so the impact of the associations is necessarily limited. In fact, I would like to tackle the issue of representation of migrants within the larger council, [rather than the issue of migrants' representations in policy-making fora in which the council is involved]. (Activist, Migrant Association, Naples, 2006)

In Naples, the main obstacle faced by associations, according to some interviewees, is the economic problems encountered in starting the project. On the one hand, due to the difficult economic area in which they work, migrants' associations cannot find and use the resources to invest in the political process. On the other hand, it is necessary to prove at least two years of activity before they have access to public funding. The first years therefore involve the personal unpaid efforts of members, and this makes it difficult to develop professional skills. That is how a representative of a migrants' association sums it up:

> ... [W]e as associations try to ask [for funding] but then the institutions ask absurd things. You can't do anything if you are not registered in their database—this in itself requires two years of activity. For a migrants' association it means that you then become their spokesperson and are legitimated to be involved in management activities ... After you have registered an association you can do something but they do not help you financially to ensure the survival of your association. (Activist, Migrant Association, Naples, 2006)

Compared with the autochthonous associations, migrants' associations are in a weak position. Not being able to consolidate, it is very difficult for the associations to take part in procurement and tenders. The projects and services available in the sector of migrants' integration are mainly managed by small- and medium-sized Italian associations which are strong, cooperative enterprises that are capable of acquiring economic resources. This opinion was expressed by several interviewees:

> In the end, a closed circuit is created whereby the approved projects belong to the same associations—it's no good that everything is concentrated among two big cooperatives whose names I won't tell, but they are linked to two names who have very personal friendship relations. They belong to managers and councilors who have a link inside the association and therefore their projects get approval. They are always at the top of the list of fully funded projects, whereas everybody else has a 50 percent cut of their funding. (Activist, Trade Union representative, Naples, 2006)

> Some voluntary associations are very strong because they have a large budget. They are the ones who always win project funding; they have friends ... but they need to have a migrant association that provides the 'ethnic touch' ... They do not bid for a project where the migrants' association is a partner with equal dignity. (Activist, Migrant Association, Naples, 2006)

Another serious problem is the lack of representativeness. This is because migrants' associations took on the worst aspects of associationism in Italy—it is as simple as that. The regional consultative body (Consulta) is an institutional place where at the beginning, migrants' representation was accepted to try to have a grip on the problems and then to try to involve them. In the last four or five years, however, we have found basic inadequacies in their approach to problems:

> That is to say, any representative of any association will find an idiosyncratic way to represent migrants *vis-à-vis* state institutions in order to bring the solutions identified by institutions to migrants. Migrant associations do not have any

> ability to formulate proposals. They are merely exploited by Italian associations in order to win public tenders and work. (Activist, Migrant Association, Naples, 2006)

Interaction with Service Provider

Analysis shows that immigrants' associations in both cities have contacts with service delivery health institutions, in particular during the initial phase of the political process: Services recognized by institutions as more profitable (formation, diffusion of information, cultural and linguistic mediation) are often delegated to immigrants' multiethnic cooperatives, with which the local health unit makes single agreements.

In both towns it is commonly thought that the main tool to facilitate integration processes is cultural mediation, which is an instrument to improve interpersonal closeness and reciprocal knowledge:

> In some contexts, without mediation, which in many cases means simply language translating, we could not have done what we did. This is also because, over time, cultural mediation, especially when done by people who possess good professional skills, is of great help not only to the operator in his dialogue with customers, but also because the cultural mediator can inform the operator about the cultural background of customers, and therefore improve the ability of the operator to understand different cultures. (Health worker, Trento, 2006)

However, the role of the cultural mediator, as the interviews reveal, has some limits in its function of community representative:

> … [W]hat matters is whether you are a permanent worker or not, because if you are permanent this is what gives you a voice in decision-making processes. The position of migrants helping on a part-time basis is absolutely marginal because for juridical reasons the majority of them, lacking Italian citizenship, can't be employed permanently, so they can't be dependent workers of a structure such as the NHS. Most of them work as freelance or for cooperatives of mediators, just delivering a service decided by other people, with their times and conditions, actually often more passing them the buck than introducing them in a real framework of intercultural mediation. (Researcher, University of Reggio Emilia, Bologna, 2006)

> Mediators are part of the team and they are often consulted; they have a certain weight but they don't have an institutional, official weight. I think that the authority system must remain the ordinary one; it is mediators and others, social anthropologists, etcetera, who have to change the mentality of managers. A mediator is a consultant; it isn't he who decides, he can't decide. Many times the idea of the mediator is taken as the rule [interviewer: 'And does he become

> bearer of requests as well?'] Sometimes yes, because he proposes smart solutions that simplify everyone's life, avoiding conflicts, difficulties, etcetera. But in the end we are back there. It's unlikely that there are two parallel powers; if the head physician must decide about health, he has to assume all the reasons, but it can't be that he decides and for example the mediator says: 'No, this is unacceptable'. (President of Italian Society of Medical Anthropology, University of Perugia, 2006)

To summarize the Italian case, one notes the prominence of the service delivery role versus the advocacy or policy-shaping role; the reliance for advocacy functions on professionals rather than migrant experts or social movement activists.

Conclusions

This chapter has illustrated the manifold functions that civil society can play in the health field. It has also illustrated: how these functions are often not satisfactorily played; how their role is discontinuous in time and space according to the vagaries of the dominant political color at different levels of government; the type of resources alternately made available and denied over time; and the general configuration of the associational field in different locations. In general terms, civil society can be utilized to several different ends: to address policy-makers' information deficit, as well as their need to aggregate interests; to formulate efficient and accepted policies, and to monitor outcomes; to help with implementation; to help policy-makers approach crises in a coherent manner; to enrich decision-making with new policy ideas; and to spur collective processes of policy learning. All these areas can benefit from the direct input of civil society groups. This also applies to migrant organizations, as they can in principle address all of these goals. This is, however, dependent upon their reception by the political establishment at various levels of governance. We will now review the main variables that structure these processes of exchange between policy-makers and civil society to identify what general lessons we can learn from our comparison.

The opportunities for political participation vary significantly in our countries according to two main variables: the societal establishment of the migrant community and the overall political environment in which they make their claims. In this respect, the difference between Canada and the two European case studies is evident: Canada's endorsement of multiculturalism has created a political culture in which civil society advocacy of migrant and minority groups is expected and institutionally encouraged. Although governed by a strong universalistic rationale, the health care system is not exempt from this political sense of entitlement. In contrast, in Germany and Italy this form of advocacy is widely perceived to be a genuine threat to the integrity of universal health service provision and migrants can voice their concerns primarily through established political channels. As was particularly manifest in the Italian case, if voice was given to migrants, it was through institutional channels of established Italian civil society organizations. In addition, migrant groups cannot rely on sources of public funding to sustain their activities; rather, they are often openly discouraged from engaging in politics as the spokesperson of a particular cultural group.

In Italy, the frequent lack of citizenship makes the migrant population particularly weak *vis-à-vis* the political process, as non-voter migrants are weakly represented in institutionalized politics. In addition, Italy, like other Mediterranean countries, has a fragmented migrant population characterized by its extremely diverse geographical, ethnic and religious background, which further weakens its ability to find internal representatives. Often differences are perceived to be relevant to the point that migrant communities do not accept individuals from other communities as representatives even when there are some linguistic and religious similarities. Thus, reliance on external experts from civil society becomes a necessity which inevitably results in a limited informational contribution. In other countries such as Canada this is less the case, making not only the informational contribution, but also the aggregative contribution of civil society more relevant.

Furthermore, the legal regulation and decision-making structures in the health care system, as well as funding opportunities for migrant associations, determine the location of advocacy efforts. When, for instance in Italy, a change of government brought a notably less migrant-friendly government, migrant associations started to redirect their efforts at the local level. In Germany, there is a striking gap between the national discourse on political inclusion and the practices at lower levels of governance and health care provision. Opportunities for migrant associations vary considerably at this local level. Thus, dynamics of venue-shopping typically characterize the advocacy efforts of pro-migrant associations and demonstrate their political skills. However, these differ across locations. If overall the local and regional levels offer a better terrain for pro-migrant advocacy, notable differences among the case studies were observed. In Leipzig and Naples, state and region were hardly involved, whilst more public involvement was manifest in Bremen and Trento. Involvement, however, has not necessarily proven to be a guarantee of effectiveness. As the Italian case demonstrates, there are typically different policy styles between the left and the right. Low levels of participation occur during right-wing governments, but the "hyper-participation" noted by, for instance, Italian activists during center-left governments could produce a confusing and ineffective array of overlapping initiatives, endless and inconclusive meetings, a cacophony of voices and decision-making blockages. This brings to the fore the issue of representation.

Policy-makers often ask whether their associational counterpart is representative of their base, and often doubt that it is. Often, migrant associations are led by "ethnic brokers" who claim to represent the diverse needs and identifications of its members, a claim that can run the risk of being based more on the leaders interest in political power than on the actual needs and interests of its members (Baumann 1999). Yet, what we have is a certain reluctance on the side of governments to include migrant associations on the level of equal representation instead of reducing them to an alibi for symbolic multiculturalism or as providing an "ethnic touch." Both aspects lead in some cases to distrust and unwillingness to grant influence and resources. This emerges, for instance, in the case of the previously-mentioned Canadian working group on the health of migrants, which was viewed as neither representing "migrant communities," nor able to report to the Minister of Health. As a loose group consisting of public health experts, it was consulted as a source of knowledge but not as a channel of representation. Similarly, as noted in Italy, the level of representation of associations is doubted by policy-makers because Italian associations involved in the sector are mainly Italian pro-migrant groups instead of migrant associations staffed by migrants. Therefore, their representativeness is openly questioned or only indirectly accepted as mediated by forms of representation that are shaped by non-migrant groups and institutional channels. If the fact that the involvement of some prestigious doctors grants legitimacy—and we have seen this in the case of Germany as well—the relative absence of migrants detracts from their potential to exert policy impact.

Thus, in terms of general participation, one notes that overall pro-migrant health associationism is generally often weak. Dynamics of internal competition for resources limit networking strategies and often engender rivalry, as both the German and the Italian cases have demonstrated. This was particularly clear in the cases of Naples and Bremen, where extreme competition limited the effectiveness of the associational field.

Moving from the structure of the field of political participation to the specific functions played by associations, one notes the centrality of service delivery. This is an area in which political approaches from the left and from the right can be combined. For the left, civil society-mediated service delivery for migrants constitutes an opportunity not only for a better implementation of policies, but also provides an opportunity to support migrant communities by fostering their economic and social equality. For the right it means decreasing the role of the state in society. However, advocacy functions are generally not welcomed in a world that increasingly sees migrants as a security threat. Especially when connected to demands for increased social and political citizenship, the advocacy of migrant organizations appears often irrelevant and possibly even unwelcome, particularly to components of the political right. To the extent that advocacy is accepted, we identified a specific role for medical professionals. As we showed in each case study, their societal legitimacy (based in their generally high social standing, image of technical competence and implicit role of guarantors of general health) provides them with a higher level of credibility in their advocacy roles.

Finally, it should be noted that both issues of legitimacy of the migrants' community and its ability to institutionalize channels of advocacy and of service delivery are dependent upon general economic trends. From this perspective the financial crisis of 2008 has altered the situation radically by increasingly differentiating the case of Italy and of Germany. While Italy has witnessed absence of economic growth for over a decade, the aftermath of the financial crisis has been particularly harsh on weak groups of the population which have faced a substantial decline in opportunities for jobs and a decline in local-level public services in housing, transportation and health. This has impacted the health role of migrant associations undermining the availability of time of volunteers, the amount of public resources available for their service-delivery roles and even their political legitimacy which declines in a period in which migrants are increasingly perceived as competitors for the appropriation of public resources. Germany in comparison withstood the crisis more effectively and continued to grow. Thus even while implementing a program of budgetary cuts in the public sector, it did not undermine the legitimacy and resources of migrant associations to the same extent as in Italy.

Chapter 4
Barriers in Access to Care

Saime Ozcurumez, Lloy Wylie, Giulia Bigot and Rika Dauth[1]

Identifying the barriers in accessing health care is a central component of examining the "success" of strategies for inclusion of migrants in the health care system. These barriers provide at least three important indicators about the interaction between minority groups and the health care system. First, they provide examples of how the legal regulations concerning cultural communities and migrants are implemented in practice. Second, these barriers indicate how the system frames the accommodation of diversity or multiculturalism. Our interviews provide insight into differences between how those working in the health care system and those in pro-migrant groups perceive the challenges of improving access to services. Third, identifying different perspectives on the access barriers demonstrates the value for dialogue between migrant groups and the system in developing access strategies, as opposed to unilateral, top-down approaches that may not be aware of key issues identified by migrants.

The data from the six cities in the three countries display strikingly similar accounts of barriers to access in the respective health care systems. Although there are more health programs for migrants in Canadian cities, barriers identified in Italy and Germany are also observed in Canada. In general migrant associations, program managers and service providers all identified common challenges and expressed concern that migrants have unequal access. Respondents stated that there were vast differences in access to care, citing matters such as geographic region (where people reside and where they access services), peoples' national or ethnic background, and varying concepts of health, socio-economic status, educational background, official language proficiency, legal status, gender and migration history. The variations in access also present a diversity of opinions on how access is viewed by different groups, depending on their relationship to the health care system (health care practitioners, policy-makers, migrant advocacy groups), and the characteristics of migrant communities (that is the size and duration of stay in the receiving country). The data characterizing the nature of access in the three cases compares and contrasts the barriers to access which emerge in the six cities in Canada, Germany and Italy. The argument in this chapter is that despite main differences in the overall governance of the health care systems in the three different countries, the challenges and barriers to accommodating cultural diversity show striking similarities.

1 The co-authors of the book were also involved in drafting chapters 4 and 5.

Knowledge of Services

A significant barrier noted in all three countries, and seen as an explanation for the limited use of services is the lack of knowledge that immigrants have about the health care system, how it works and what services they have a right to access. In Montreal it was expressed that immigrants or refugees "come here and they don't know the ropes, they don't know the rules of the game" (representative, migrant association, Montreal, 2006). And similarly in Bremen it was noted that "There are many, many migrants who have no idea how things work here in Germany, how many institutions are there" (social worker in a hospital, Russian-speaking addictions services, Bremen, 2007).

One reason identified for the lack of knowledge of the health care system is that many immigrants do not have experience with welfare state models of service access (as in Canada and Italy) or the German pluralist model. As one Canadian health care provider noted, many immigrants have different conceptions and expectations about health services and institutions:

> We have people coming from refugee camps or displaced areas where they have not necessarily experienced the type of health system that we have. This concept of family doctors and having appointments and being on time to be seen does not necessarily hold true for this population, not at least at the beginning because they are totally unfamiliar. In refugee camps most services are drop-in, people wait for a long time and are not used to seeing a doctor and they might just see a nurse or the promoter because that's all they have there … So the lack of knowledge of the system is very important at that patient level. (Doctor, hospital clinic, Vancouver, 2008)

In Leipzig it was noted that migrants often face difficulties with the mechanisms, norms and regulations of the health care system in Germany:

> Our health system is performing highly efficiently but can seem quite complicated, if you come from a country where you have a government based medical care. Those sometimes have a poor quality of supplies, but are more simple to convey and more comprehensible to the citizens. Our pluralist system, however, is quite incomprehensible. (State Manager of the Health Insurance Fund, Leipzig, 2007)

It was also expressed that the lack of education among immigrants is a constraint for access, particularly in Germany and Italy. The German health system, with its reliance on written information about health conditions and treatments, is geared toward literate, educated patients and thus excludes non-literate patients with low educational levels. There is often a lack of interpreters to allow staff to provide information on specific conditions or on the health care system to migrant patients and/or their families that lack German language skills. In addition, without the

German literacy skills to read the materials provided, migrant patients do not have access to understandable information on their condition. In Germany it was also noted that knowledge of health services does not reach those with low or very limited educational levels, even if this information is translated into the dominant migrant languages in written format:

> I know many who have not attended schools here … They have no relation towards papers and so on, information leaflets. They don't know that. You give it to them and they throw it away. But if you sit down and explain to them, they understand! (Midwife, Bremen, 2007)

Lack of knowledge about the health care system is directly associated with the underuse of services. Gaps in knowledge are attributed to two main factors. First, there is a lack of agreement on who is responsible for ensuring that information on the health care system is communicated to migrants. Second, problems originate from the lack of institutionalized practices to address needs arising from diversity, particularly in the German health system.

In Italy, there is significant variation of knowledge of the health care system among immigrants, with some very aware while others have no knowledge about how the system works and the services available to them. The perception of the interviewees, both at the national and local levels, suggests that the differences in access to health services reflect many factors that contribute to the variation in knowledge of the health system, including migrants' characteristics, such as country of origin, knowledge of the destination country, duration of their stay, their motives for migration and their proficiency in the official languages. Nonetheless the data from the interviews in Italy highlight two main factors that contribute to knowledge of and access to health care services. First, the economic situation of the migrant is a key determinant of how they relate to the health care system, as exemplified by the following quote:

> The real problem is the lack of economic means. If I am a highly trained immigrant of Chinese descent who is managing a chain of Chinese restaurants in the North of Italy, I am sorry, but of what use is a clinic for foreign women? The real discrimination is at the level of economic achievement and is related to the awareness of how to get information that helps you to take care of yourself and your health. This is discriminatory. (Health care manager, Trento, 2007)

Second, the extent to which migrants make use of their community network for accessing knowledge on the health care system and the services is another important factor shaping access of the services. The social capital of migrants (that is community networks) and how they use it are decisive in determining the knowledge and use of health care services. Therefore, both transnational experience and the presence of social networks greatly impact migrants' settlement practices (Castles and Miller 2003; Faist and Ozveren 2004; Jordan and Duvell 2003; Levitt 2009).

Our data from the three countries confirms the variation in social capital among different migrants, its impact and how health care services are accessed. First, migrants might have moved to a location where members from their community are few in number. Therefore the possibility of accessing a pre-existing social network is low or absent, limiting support they receive from their community about the health care system. Second, although the number of community members might be large, they might not be as organized and might lack economic resources, therefore limiting the efficiency of their support network. As suggested in the following quotes by a consultant from a pro-migrant doctors' association and a service provider: "There are communities that have ways of getting together spontaneously and channeling their claims towards access to services" (pro-migrant doctor, 2006).

> Why does an immigrant opt for a particular country? Very often this decision is based on a pre-existing social network that helps in the settlement process; hence this is the social network that in the end also determines access to health services. This is because whoever came first, obviously knows already how the system works, which are the access points and modes of accessing the health care system. So if there is already a strong reference community, it is more likely that this group will have easier access. (Doctors without Borders, Milan, 2007)

> There are those from the East, Ukraine or Moldova, who have been here for a year or two but have such a strong social network because of their sister, mother, or simply friends, that they know more than we do and who succeed in dealing with the health services in a much better way than we would be able to do by directing them in the right direction. But then there are those from Bangladesh, less from India who are completely incapable of finding their way through the health care system. This is because if the husbands are not around they cannot accomplish anything. Here we often have the husbands but not the wives. We ask with resolve for the wives to come, but they rarely do. They are accompanied by their husbands every time and for everything, this means for the gynecologist, the pediatrician, to have an analysis done, etc. For everything they need to be accompanied. In contrast, the North Africans from Morocco, Tunisia and Algeria, which is one of our more established minorities, have developed a good degree of autonomy over the years. However, not all of them have this (autonomy) because while being here for many years they often do not speak Italian at all; yet they might have a friend, a neighbor. Hence the social network seems to be the key to success when it comes to access. (Service provider, Trento, 2006)

The findings across all cases suggest that the cultural community to which the individual belongs can shape knowledge about and access to the health care system, and therefore acts as a "mediator" which might or might not "facilitate" service knowledge and use.

It should be noted that lack of information about the health care system is not only a problem that affects migrants. For example, the Italian public sector is generally organized through a set of often obscure and byzantine bureaucratic norms, which affect the entire population (Geraci et al. 2010). However, the Italian population is often able to circumvent the limitations of this system through informal or even corrupt access to the resources of the system and through indirectly acquired information from personal networks. Migrants face the additional problem of sparse and information-poor networks which translate into limitations of access in a bureaucratic and legalistic system that creates barriers for those with low levels of education and social capital.

Differential Use of Health Care Services

Variations in access among immigrants and across the health system itself make it difficult to present a definitive statement about the level and quality of access to health care services, as exemplified in the following quote:

> the major stumbling block is that the whole thing is so haphazard … You got some very good situations, some middle of the road and some real horror stories. So, you got a whole spectrum of possible answers, and it's all left to local people to somehow organize themselves to get the service that they need. (Representative, Migrant Association, Montreal, 2006)

A program manager made a similar statement, noting that:

> Differences in treatment that exist between different groups, again, I think it very much depends on any individual's ability to negotiate equitable care with their provider. (Program manager, hospital, Vancouver, 2006)

In all three countries there are similar trends regarding how immigrants access health care services. All cases show a lower use of services in general, but particularly so for preventive programs, meaning that immigrants are more likely to not receive preventive or early intervention, instead accessing care at a later stage of illness. This is related to the lack of knowledge about services and also to not having a family doctor that can monitor their health and guide them to additional health services. In Canada it was noted by both program managers and service providers that often migrants come to the health care system in worse health, usually through the emergency departments, rather than to a family doctor, which many do not have. An interviewee in Vancouver noted that "generally it seems that there are delays in presenting for care, people present more often in emergency wards" (program manager, hospital, Vancouver, 2006).

Similar trends are noted in Germany, with migrant groups using emergency care much more than other services, and a significant lack of use of prevention or early intervention programs. The likelihood that immigrants arrive in advanced stages of an illness at a medical facility is therefore much higher compared to the native-born population. In Germany the interviewees attributed such underutilization to a lack of health focused organizations among immigrant groups such as breast cancer or diabetes self-help groups, which are more common in Canada. An interesting point is that the underutilization of preventive services is present in both cases with or without the migrant health focused self-help groups. In Italy preventive care is also underutilized by immigrant communities, who instead access health care services under more urgent circumstances such as when they are seriously ill or in advanced stages of pregnancy. Many migrant associations try to address this problem by providing their clients with information on health services, and particularly on how to find a family doctor. For example an association of the Chinese community in Montreal provides lists of Mandarin-speaking family doctors who may accept new patients. Such examples from all three cases attest to the critical role of the social networks among established migrants on facilitating access to the health care system.

In Canada the awareness of the need for accessing preventive services has increased for those who participate in the self-help groups. Some migrants and their representatives in Germany point to significant care gaps within health services in relation to the needs of migrants and refugees. Although the Bremen-based association Refugio is among the few associations that offer mental health care for victims of torture, Germany generally lacks programs for asylum-seekers in the field of mental health. In Leipzig and many other cities such programs are absent, as noted by the interviewees in a care institution: "It is a rather a marginal issue, in the case of war-trauma for example, we have no experience with treatments" (Director of the children and youth advisory board Kaktus e.V., Leipzig, 2007). Similarly in Canada it was also mentioned by a migrant association in Montreal that there are no services for survivors of war and torture, despite the significant need. Therefore, the lack of these services suggests that immigrants may not access the specialized services they need since the system does not even acknowledge those special treatment needs.

In general, the use of mental health services, for example, was lower for immigrants when compared to the native-born population in Germany, Italy and Canada. In Germany it is noted that immigrants are overrepresented in the institutionalized care of mental health services while ambulatory care is accessed less. The gap is explained by late intervention as a result of a lack of availability of migrant-specific ambulatory care (in particular of mother language services) combined with cultural taboos on mental health care. Immigrants are more likely to intervene at a later stage of their mental problems, so, by the time they access the services, they already have reached a more advanced stage that could have been prevented by earlier intervention. In Canada it was similarly noted that many immigrants were apprehensive about using mental health services because of the stigma attached to it. In addition, a representative from a migrant association explained that the mental health of immigrants is not seen as a priority in health planning in Montreal, despite the well-known mental and emotional stress that migration puts on people.

In Italy, the interviewees underlined that lack of knowledge about the system leads to inappropriate use of services where emergency care is the main point of access to health services. Despite long line-ups, services are provided for all—regular or irregular migrants and at all hours—without asking too many questions. In this way, sparse information often leads to an overcrowding of health care facilities and misunderstandings with service providers.

> Women who do not speak Italian, Arab, Macedonian or Albanian from Kosovo, waiting for the return of their men from work would go there in the evening. The emergency room has always been busy, also on Saturdays and Sundays after five or six pm. And they couldn't understand why, if every day there is a general practitioner on duty, for every urgent need you can go there. Instead even for an earache you go to the emergency room because it's the only way. I feel sick, then I go to the emergency room. Even if things have changed, that's how we are. (AMIC 2006)[2]

Another interviewee in Trento notes that the inadequate use of health care services creates pressures on the health care system in that there is an excess use of emergency services in cases

> that would not warrant an emergency solution, an urgent access to emergency services, or the immediate recourse to emergency treatment. This overloads our system with an enormous amount of requests for treatment that very often could have been taken care of by other means. (Trade Union, Rome, 2007)

In the case of regular immigrants who may enjoy the same rights as Italians, the interviewees underlined that the differences in the use of services could rather be attributed to different cultural conceptions of health and the body (for instance in prevention programs, in prenatal courses and so on) by different cultural groups. For instance in Trento it was noted that: "Women coming from Eastern Europe, they have a more relaxed and confident relationship to dealing with services in the health care system, whereas women from the Maghreb or Pakistan have a far more complicated relationship" (Trade Union, Rome, 2007). In Naples a medical doctor stated:

> The Chinese community is the most reserved when it comes to the encounter with our services and it is not by accident that this group, I imagine, is at highest

2 AMIC is the association of intercultural mediators formed in Trento in November 2002. See www.associazioneamic.it.

> risk. From various sets of data that we have, Chinese women are the strongest group among those who commit suicide. The group that has less difficulty with our health system—some of the difficulties that all have—are women from Eastern Europe where in all likelihood the approach to the body is very similar to ours. (Medical doctor, Naples, 2007)

Location "Matters" for Access

The availability of services specifically oriented to the needs of immigrants varies significantly by location. In Vancouver it was noted that the clinic specifically oriented to migrants was located in the center of the city, while many recently arrived migrants are moving into communities in the suburban areas where housing is more affordable. In some of the outlying areas where immigrants are settling, the services and infrastructure are not in place for meeting the health needs of immigrant communities, such as access to immigrant settlement agencies, interpreter services or staff with training in culturally competent care. Yet respondents in both Vancouver and Montreal noted that in some respects this made the service planners neglect the need to adapt services in other locations with a smaller presence of culturally diverse communities. This has led to significant variation in experience with the health care system depending on where people live, as described by a migrant association representative, who noted "complete barriers to anything to do with cultural access" in areas outside of the urban centers (representative, Migrant Association, Vancouver, 2006).

In Germany the almost non-existent availability of mother language services in most cities and outside of city centers was also noted as a constraint for access: "Two and a half hours to go and two and a half hours to come back for 45 minutes' therapy makes people fail to come, though the need is very high" (social worker, mental hospital, Bremen, 2007). It was also noted that service providers try to direct non-German patients to services that are more equipped for serving those communities: "Foreign patients appear in university hospitals disproportionately more often, because they are burdens or less favorable than an average German patient for established doctors in the ambulances due to language barriers, so those patients often are referenced to university walk-in clinics" (member, Medical Board of the University Hospital of Leipzig, 2007). Such a finding confirms the overwhelming use of emergency services by migrants rather than preventive services.

In Italy the interviews also indicate that there are notable differences in the extent to which the health system welcomes migrant patients across different locations, despite norms of inclusiveness as the main operating principle for the system as a whole. The following statements by service providers attest to this observation: "At the normative level I think that there is an unanimous feeling that our approach is very favorable, very much avant-garde if you want. However at the operational level there are, as always, blank spots … As far as I am aware of there is still a lot of variation at the level of applying these norms" (service provider, Trento, 2006). Within the health care system "there are those who interpret the norms in a more inclusive way and those who tend to apply them in more exclusive fashion" (service provider, Naples, 2006). Therefore the observation is that there is a gap between norms of inclusiveness and practices of exclusiveness in some parts of the system. All the interviews indicate that this gap needs to be narrowed and/or eliminated in order to facilitate de facto access to the health care system, particularly in the Italian and Canadian cases.

There are also structural regional differences in access to care that are more specifically linked to economic issues: some regions are wealthier and allocate more funds in mediation services, specific services such as mental health or prenatal courses. Poorer regions have fewer funds available for those services or do not have those services at all, which results in poorer quality of services for immigrants and non-immigrants alike. The findings of all the cases suggest that there is a gap between the promises and the services of the health care system (for example when comparing the legal commitments in the Canadian and Italian cases vs. the practice in the health care system). Additionally service provision varies across the different cities and in fact among different neighborhoods in the same city. For example a migrant living in a high migrant density neighborhood has more chances of accessing health care services compared to a migrant who lives in a low migrant density neighborhood. This situation is currently further deteriorating as a consequence of the process of health regional decentralization. As Geraci points out:

> The current progressive administrative and political decentralization is producing an extreme heterogeneity of health provisions on the national territory, which is due to a very variable level of attention of public service administrations on the local level. This can then determine inequalities in access to services, and variations in the state of health of the migrant population of different localities. (Geraci et al. 2010. 5)

Thus, to summarize, migrants' access to health in Italy is unequally distributed according to a wide set of variables, which include class, ethnicity, network extension and resources, and region of residence. In Italy access is firstly de facto more limited because cultural mediation as a facilitating factor is hindered by the multi-provenance background of Italian migration. This limits the possibility to express focused demands and representative advocacy. Still, there are several urban neighborhoods with a high concentration of single-language groups such as the Arabs in many Italian cities, or the South American community in Genoa.

Secondly, while access is facilitated by migrant workers in the health service, hiring staff with a migration background is hindered by (a) the general low educational level and high geographical mobility of Italian migrants; and (b) the non-acceptance of foreign degrees. However, this situation is rapidly changing as a more integrated and linguistically competent second and third generation of migrant population is emerging and practicing as health professionals.

In addition to these general factors, there are also political factors and factors pertaining to internal territorial differences. In terms of internal differences, the strong North–South divide makes access generally more difficult in the South due to a multi-sector weak state capacity (see Geraci et al. 2010: 41). As for political factors, the sector is partly regulated at the national level and partly at the regional level. There are relevant disparities between different regions according to their political perspectives. Center-right regions tend to see immigration as a security problem and health as an issue area in which human rights, the health concerns of the native population, and the spending priorities of the state conflict. Thus one tends to find less of a focus on the health of migrants than in regions ruled by center-left coalitions. In this context, the recent attempt by the center-right government to limit the right of health providers not to report irregular migrants to the authorities tends to have a discouraging impact on access to services. Typically regions of central Italy with a strong tradition of center-left local governments tend to have regional health plans that pay more attention to migrants (see map 5 in Geraci et al. 2010: 42).

Access to policy developments is improving as migrants' associations are learning advocacy skills from Italian associations. As evidenced in the following quote, the association of cultural mediators in Trento recognizes the contribution of the mainly Italian association Gruppi Regionali Immigrazione e Salute (GRIS or "Regional Groups on Immigration and Health") in establishing its presence:

> We come from countries in which associations are not very present. So in forming associations we needed someone who showed us the way … So we were offered support during our first year. We learned how to do consultancies, how to prepare a statute, and so on. (AMIC 2005)

However, even in this case territorial differences remain crucial as the third sector is more resourced, more numerous and more skilled in the North.

Group-Specific Differences in Access to Care

In Vancouver and Montreal a common theme was that access varied across cultural groups. Yet the framing of this unequal access was quite different in the two locations. In Vancouver the main difference in access to care was based on questions of critical mass in population numbers and length of time the community had been using the system. Communities with larger numbers and longer histories in Canada have better access than people from newer waves of immigration. Program managers and community liaison personnel in Vancouver discussed the importance of these factors in access to care:

> numbers probably create better access. So, some of the larger groups—it's Cantonese, Mandarin and Punjabi in Vancouver and surrounding areas. So I think that those groups probably tend to have more voice. And because of the numbers, we also have more resources. So there are more Cantonese speakers who are also fluent English speakers, who will then take the initiative to go and get proper training at Vancouver Community College, and so that impacts that. There are what we call languages of lesser diffusion … where they're having to rely on resources that are not as well trained, maybe not as accessible, so maybe appointments have to be changed—so it does change, from group to group. (Program manager, translation services, Vancouver, 2006)

There is a clear understanding among all interviewees in Bremen that groups with a larger and more established community fare better in accessing health services. This was demonstrated by the link between size of the community and greater network density, self-help potential and familiarity due to longer periods of stay. For example, this service provider notes that: "Turks are a specific group here and I have a feeling that they have the best conditions, because they all know each other. People from other countries who do not belong to this ethnic group have less chances" (psychologist, Bremen, 2006). Members of the second or third generation of larger groups show a higher presence as professionals in the health care sector and for matters of cultural and mother language competence can provide better services for their community. The presence of health care providers from a variety of migrant communities is expected to increase the probability of accessing the system and with better means.

Groups that had been in Vancouver for a shorter period of time, such as refugees, or people coming from war-torn regions, had worse access, compared to those who had been residing there longer. Both of these groups were usually fewer in number and consisted of people speaking "languages of lesser diffusion," who often have greater and varied health care needs. It was also noted by a Vancouver program manager that the care provided to certain communities, while they are accessible, may not be appropriate for their needs, based on the fact that services are designed without their particular needs in mind:

> For example HIV, AIDS. Clearly that's a condition that affects more people from Africa. And so, are the HIV services accessible? Probably they are. You could get an interpreter and go to one. Would it be appropriate? Not likely, because it would be the services developed by and for Caucasian, middle-class, men, mostly, and we get a lot of HIV women, right? Black, African women. (Diversity program manager, hospital, Vancouver, 2006)

In Montreal, the discussion about racism and discrimination in the system was prevalent among many of the respondents, who noted that European immigrants in Canada fare much better in terms of access to care:

> The further away you get from the European culture, the further you get towards, like say, Africa or Asia, groups that are very recent, that do not share the same values as the European traditional Canadian majority, then the resources will not be there. So health care will not be as good. So again, it has a lot to do with the time factor, and it has to do with cultural prejudices that are built into the way that Quebec and Canada perceive the population. (Representative, Migrant Association, Montreal, 2006)

In Germany, some respondents assess group identity and access by how prepared institutions are for providing migrant-specific care, as seen in this quote: "Depending on the language, some people are better taken care of and some worse. We have our channels: Russian, Turkish, a social worker from the neighboring clinic speaks Russian" (hospital director, Bremen, 2007). This perspective shifts the focus away from the capacity of the migrant person or group, such as lack of language skills, as the barriers to health care access, to the deficiencies in the institutional setting, such as which languages are used for interpretation to facilitate access. Therefore the migrant-friendliness of a hospital is framed as a key determinant for shaping access.

In the German context, national background is often used as a reference point to determine the capacity of a migrant to integrate. For example, migrants from the CIS (Commonwealth of Independent States) are seen as having less capacity to integrate when compared to migrants with a Turkish background, due to lack of a social network. Other quotes confirm the low "integration potential" among migrants from the CIS, but apply a different explanatory pattern: "The Russian speaking is not covered. Ethnic Germans were a group one had not prepared for" (psychologist, Bremen, 2007). This discourse frames the health care system as deficient in the efforts to accommodate diversity, which leads to unequal access. The German case also demonstrates the ethnic or cultural identity markers as part of the prejudice built into the health care system, with certain migrant communities assumed to be predisposed to specific disorders; the Polish and the Russians are seen as prone to alcoholism, while the Turks are prone to psychiatric problems.

Some interviewees linked certain cultural groups with lower levels of education and socio-economic status. In these cases, class and ethnicity combined determine prospects for access:

> Somebody from the Iranian middle class will easily find access to this society, even to the health care system then somebody who comes from Kurdistan and is illiterate. The threshold for Kurds is much higher as they come from a milieu where they have not visited schools and cannot imagine how to approach Germans in order to access care. (Psychotherapist, Migrant Association, Bremen, 2007)

In Leipzig the interviewees repeatedly presume that access depends on the degree to which the health care system of the migrant's country of origin is similar to the

German one. "It is the experience with the health care sector of the country of origin that makes the difference. I think that for example migrants from the USA have a better access to our health care system because the health supply is probably similar to ours and psychotherapists are commonly well known" (Director of the child and youth advisory board Kaktus e.V., Leipzig, 2007). The native language of the migrant is also cited as one of the significant variables determining access to the health care system. The more rarely the native language of the migrant is used, the more difficulties appear with access to the health care system: "It is difficult, if there is somebody from Africa, who is only speaking a particular dialect but neither English nor German. In this case it would be almost impossible to give him certain advices" (State manager of the health insurance fund, Leipzig, 2007).

Several interviewees mentioned that the prospects for access improve if there are medical staff with a similar migration background. For example, although Vietnamese people have been present in Leipzig for a very long time and constitute the largest group of migrants in Leipzig there exists only one Vietnamese doctor while there are many professional medical staff from Russia or Russian speakers.

In Italy some respondents stated that discrimination was not a serious concern, as cited in the following statement: "The cases of discrimination are considered to be generally rare and related to the commonplace difficulties and structures related to a normal degree of ignorance of norms, and sometimes to a certain degree of arrogance in particular situations" (Trade Union, Rome, 2007). Moreover the cases of discrimination are cited as being anecdotal rather than generalized in the system as a whole: "It is difficult to generalize this for the immigrants. There might be situations and incidents of racism but they are attached to individual persons" (Doctors without Borders, Milan, 2007). Most of the statements also confirmed that the norm of inclusiveness was widespread in the system:

> In my opinion the health care system is a form of public service provision that is very wide/broad for all of us, be it autochthones or foreigners. The behavior of front line health care workers is really only a secondary issue. It can happen to all of us independent from where we come from. One can encounter a worker who is more or less polite; it all depends on the situation … I have never heard of anybody who had the door shut in his/her face. (Migrant Association, Trento, 2006)

Various interviewees in Italy have however pointed to cases of improper behavior toward immigrants, in particular irregular migrants, that compromises equal access and reflects an attitude shaped by prejudice. For instance there are situations in which immigrants are treated improperly and in a demeaning fashion; for example "when immigrants are immediately addressed with the 'tu' (non-polite form) which in this case is not a sign of progressive familiarity" (Trade Union, Rome, 2007).

Such statements on the system signify a common challenge across all cases. The different systems have a complex interplay of the commitment to equal treatment for all and the stereotyping of and prejudice toward different cultural groups. Therefore the commitment to equal treatment is simultaneously delimited by the emphasis on ethnic-specific problems or care needs.

Language Barriers

Language barriers are seen as the most significant barrier in health care services for immigrants. Access to interpretation services varies across location, service and language group in all three countries.

Although there was some sentiment in Germany that immigrants should be learning German, many respondents felt that the health care system itself needed to make a greater effort to address these language barriers. In Bremen, most quotes referred to language as one of the main access barriers in the absence of foreign-language based health services: "We have great difficulties to treat Polish and Russian patients, because they hardly speak German. This is also the case for other migrant groups" (social worker, hospital, Bremen, 2007).

In Germany in the 1980s and 1990s it was noted that cleaning personnel of migrant background served as translators for migrant patients trying to access hospital services. In the 2000s Bremen introduced professional translation services. The Bureau of Public Health established a translation service in 2005 which is hardly used because of the high costs involved. Instead of taking advantage of the professional translation service of the Bureau of Public Health hospitals have established "internal translation pools." These pools consist of lists of staff with a migration background (mainly nurses) serving as "on call" untrained translators during their normal working hours. However the data from the interviews reveal that although these services are available, their use in the system is precarious at best. Most of the interviews cite the language barrier as a major obstacle for accessing services, as highlighted by the following remark by a psychologist working in gynecological oncology in Bremen, who notes:

> Sometimes I realize it with elderly Russian women who do not know what kind of operation is being performed on them. They ask things like: "Is the operation really over?" And then she asks, what has actually been done and one thinks that that had already been explained to her. That is a big loss, when this information just gets lost like that. (Hospital psychologist, Bremen, 2006)

Since 2005 diversity training has been offered in all Bremen hospitals with a steadily increasing demand, with some offering language courses (French and English) as well for their staff. While not being part of the officially-recognized medical colleges, nursing schools have incorporated diversity training into their curricula.[3]

3 The credit points for diversity training courses are however rather low which means the students have less incentive to take them.

One of the common focal points of diversity training in hospitals is the topic "mourning and death in diverse cultures" as staff feel particularly helpless in such contexts. Trainees generally reported that their working conditions are improving as a result of having received the training. Some hospitals have invited religious leaders to give insights on Muslim mourning rituals and sometimes training takes place in mosques. Several NGOs and welfare organizations in Bremen also offer diversity training, for example Refugio offers training for psychotherapists and translators. Three hospitals allowed doctoral students to engage in research on migrant-friendly practices in their wards.

Similar to Bremen, some hospitals in Leipzig rely on their staff with a migration background, though in a less organized way. In rare cases, when staff are not available professional translators are also utilized: "If we can get translators who work as medical staff in our hospital this is always better since they are more familiar with the facts. But if there is no other possibility we call (professional) translators" (Medical Board of the University Clinic, Leipzig, 2006).

Medical doctors in Leipzig had contradictory views on the issue of translation in terms of migrants' rights. Some argued that the "right for translation" was an issue that had to be legally enshrined, for which medical associations would be responsible, while other doctors found these rights sufficiently met already: "In fact it is already legally regulated that it is not possible to operate on a patient without his or her consent. Nevertheless he can only agree in the sense of informed consent if he understood … If he does not understand, a translator is obligatory" (Medical Board of the University Clinic, Leipzig, 2006).

The common practice of the health care sector actually diverts from legal arrangements in the sense that even if patients do not understand, translators are not used in all cases. There are several cases where patients receive treatment, including operations, without consent and without understanding the type of treatment, operation or therapy (Wesselmann and Lindemeyer 2004). While medical doctors were partly reluctant in their attitude toward legally regulating translation rights, mental health experts strongly highlighted the need for secured translation services:

> Particularly in psychiatry, translators are inevitable. Since there are no objectified examination methods, 90 percent is based on a personal or external anamnesis. You have to talk to each other. Everything else is nonsense. (Health Office, Leipzig, 2007)

In this context, practitioners with foreign language skills were frequently mentioned as a comparative advantage for health care service organizations, as they would save eventual translation costs and improve services for migrant patients.

Despite the fact that health practitioners in Leipzig generally support the use of translation services, these services are rarely used, except for emergency cases and in the absence of other means of translation such as relatives or other hospital personnel. Interviewees stressed that the few existing professional translators are not preferred, since they lack the necessary medical competence. A central reason for the lack of professional translation services lies, according to all interviewees, in the lack of financial resources due to severe financial cuts for German hospitals. Though DRGs (Diagnosis Related Groups) allocate funds for translation services hospitals set other priorities and only in rare cases use these funds for their actual purpose.

There are two basic perspectives on the issue of migrant-specific translation (cultural and linguistic) among migrant advocates in Bremen. The promoters of cultural translators view mere linguistic translation as a limitation that ignores access barriers created by "cultural difference" (Bahadir 2011). The counter-narrative critically objects to cultural translators by viewing the emphasis on culture as a practice that may reinforce stereotyping and lead to exclusion. Between 2005 and 2008 one of the welfare organizations (Paritätisches Bildungswerk) trained a group of cultural translators for the health care system and a group of unemployed migrants have been trained as community health workers (MiMi: With Migrants for Migrants). This training took place as part of a nationwide initiative in various cities organized by the Ethnomedical Centre Hannover in cooperation with the bureaus of public health. Our data indicates that it has been extremely difficult for these cultural mediators to gain employment in a system that shows no willingness to allocate or use funding for such purposes.

Migrant representatives in Leipzig consider communication as a major necessity in the context of migrants' access to health care, because migrant with little or no German skills usually face discrimination in health institutions. When there are professional translators present, it is more likely that staff abstain from discrimination. In reaction to this situation, qualifications and workshops for translators and cultural mediators in the field of medicine have been launched by the project "Health needs Communication" (Gekomm[4]—GesundheitbrauchtKommunikation), an NGO that provides translation services free of charge for migrants. Gekomm's key strategy is the assignment of cultural mediators and translators for migrant patients accessing medical institutions. Gekomm also emphasizes a high need for translators in mental health.

The policy-makers and practitioners interviewed in Bremen regarding the issue of cultural and linguistic translators were generally not well informed about existing migrant-specific structures in the health care system. The integration officer for instance assumed that the translation service offered by the bureau of public health was covered by the health insurance. Like most people we interviewed in Bremen he was also not aware that the service was hardly accessed by hospitals. He nevertheless emphasized that hospitals have improved by introducing internal translation services, whereby hospitals have begun to use doctors and nurses, rather than cleaning personnel, as translators. Most policy-makers and practitioners support a discourse in which migrants are charged with the responsibility to

4 Unfortunately funding for Gekomm was terminated and at the time of writing there are no translation services free of charge offered in Leipzig.

acquire German language skills. This responsibility would free the state and/or health care institutions from having to provide translators. Cultural translators are more or less ignored in the public discourse of policy-makers and practitioners as cultural identities are expected to dissolve in the process of integration: "Once they receive German citizenship they are Germans anyway and have adapted to German culture" (integration officer, Bremen, 2006).

Policy-makers and practitioners in Leipzig noted that due to the low demand for translators there is almost no need for professional translators in hospitals. Instead, they suggest using community translators who will be employed by the local government, thereby providing services not only in the health sector but also in official state institutions facing diversity such as the Integration Office and schools. The city of Berlin employs such community translators. They are members of migrant communities who work on a voluntary basis: "The projects where people from the community communicate into the community are the most successful, I think, because here the cultural understanding is deciding. This cannot be transmitted by somebody from outside who has in fact no access to the group" (migrant policy expert, Berlin, 2007). An example from Berlin shows that community translators can be deployed in several fields beyond the health sector such as in education or in other state institutions.

In Canada the lack of proficiency in the official languages (English and French) is viewed as the most significant barrier for using health care services. Accordingly there are various initiatives and programs for providing interpretation and translation services in both Vancouver and Montreal. In Montreal, an Interregional Bank of Interpreters (IBI) was launched in April 1993 with a mandate from the Ministry of Health and Social Services (MSSS). The IBI was created as a result of consultations carried out by the MSSS representatives focusing on different models developed in France, Switzerland and Belgium as well as studying the needs of the communities in Quebec concerning translation services. The model for interpretation services also accounted for the training of interpreters. A wide consultation with immigrants, community organizations, health practitioners and training program designers has taken place. Starting in 2000 a continuing education training program for health interpreters has been offered at the University of Montreal. The training of other (non-health) interpreters is provided by the University of Montreal and at Université du Québec à Montréal (UQAM) in inter-cultural communication and interpretation, connected with the Languages Department at the University of Montreal.

The IBI aims to have a sufficient number of interpreters covering approximately 60 languages, and they try to have a male and a female interpreter available for each language group. The objective of the program is to maintain this profession as a career and the program managers try to ensure sustained employment for translators in the program.

The IBI provides additional training to interpreters for health services including training material concerning the specific challenges such as the need to complement translation skills with knowledge about health to ensure appropriate diagnosis. The vast majority of interpreters with the IBI (90 percent) are themselves immigrants. They also work as cultural facilitators, assisting health professionals in cross-cultural communication. The IBI receives more than 100 calls per day, and provides more than 20,000 hours of interpretation per year, with about 90 percent of this for services in Montreal. The IBI provides their services to health establishments, schools and public institutions in the health and social services network. They also provide guide materials for service providers on working with interpreters:

> Interpretation in the health sector is different than interpretation of a conference. You are not hiding in a little booth. You don't have a colleague to whisper words to you. You are sometimes very close to the client. If you are in a small community, then, everyone knows each other. So how do you manage this stress, this pressure? So that's part of the training that we provide. (Program manager, translation services, Montreal, 2006)

One drawback about the interpretation services that the health professionals raise is that there should be a standardized national accreditation process, with professional recognition and equitable salaries, which as yet does not exist.

Before the IBI, and even after it had been established, various hospitals in Quebec use interpreters with whom they have established connections, particularly for unplanned interpretation, as expressed by one program manager as:

> in cases of doubt … it's recommended that an interpreter be present. And sometimes the family might get offended, because they say, you know, I understand English, or French or whatever. And [what we] say to them [is that we want] to make sure that we don't make any mistakes. We want to be absolutely sure that on both sides we fully understand. (Diversity program manager, hospital, Montreal, 2006)

The same manager also highlights the significance of having interpreters who also act as cultural mediators in the following way:

> We have an interpretation service and we do about 6,000 interpretations a year. We also do screening and selecting of interpreters and training for interpreters. We do four sessions a year … And the interpreters act as cultural mediators, helping bridge the gap between family and physician or professional, helping them understand the cultural context and the practices and the customs, and to incorporate those into health care delivery. To ensure … compliance, the families are more likely to follow through on the medical plan, if their needs are understood, their beliefs are respected. At the same time, if their practices are acknowledged, they can then sometimes incorporate those practices … So it just makes for a better outcome all around. People feel more comfortable, they feel that they're connecting. (Diversity program manager, hospital, Montreal, 2006)

Similar to the case of Germany hospitals have attempted to devise informal and ad hoc arrangements to address the need for translation services. Occasionally they hire community organizations which charge lower fees than IBI or engage medical students who speak more than one language and ask them for translation services while they are working as volunteers or conducting their internships.

Overall the lack of effective communication or understanding between patients and health service providers creates significant problems. Language barriers severely reduce the quality of health care due to communication deficits. As one migrant association representative in Montreal noted: "There were cases here of false diagnoses because of incomprehension … there are also false diagnostics because of a lack of communication" (representative, Migrant Association, Montreal, 2006).

Another issue that was addressed in Italy was the lack of patience of front line workers while treating immigrants because of linguistic difficulties:

> Italy will never be able to find an appropriate response to immigration. We have witnessed immigration for quite some time now but our institutions are indifferent, hypocritical. This is because those who work in the offices are not available; they feel annoyed when immigrants speak with them and have no patience to listen to a person who does not speak Italian well. It is a form of closure that immigrants encounter, for instance when they go the hospital; as a result the immigrant always hides. (Migrant Association, Naples, 2007)

In Trento, a similar problem with language skills is cited as a barrier to access particularly affecting female migrants as noted in the following statement:

> There is a Muslim minority, mostly women, who access the health care system knowing that they do not know the language and expecting that the accompanying husband helps them with issues of access. This tells us that we need to take into account a cultural aspect and thus an aspect of family life in which the wife only acts if accompanied by the husband. We need to develop measures acknowledging that Muslim women often do not know Italian, have a low level of education and are in constant need of their husband without whom they cannot express themselves. To some degree this determines access and at the same time creates problems: Consider for instance the situation in which a woman faces intimidations related to abortion; it really changes things if this woman could come to the hospital secretly rather than having to wait until the husband comes home from work in the evening. For women from the East, this is not a problem at all. (Service provider, Trento, 2007)

It was also noted that the language is not just a barrier when speaking with care providers, as a lack of signs in hospitals also creates access barriers. In Trento and Naples, for example, another barrier is the difficulty in understanding which building to go to because the signs for directions are in Italian. Similar barriers are cited for Canada and Germany as well. For example, a program manager in Montreal noted that often patients will leave the hospital without accessing all of the services that they are there for:

> because they're afraid to ask where is the x-ray so they go round and round in the hospital and finally they get tired and they go home. Because they are afraid to be looked at as an ignorant person so they don't ask. They simply leave … 'I didn't know where to go, I was shy, I was afraid' … So they're not asking. (Program manager, hospital, Montreal, 2006)

Some interviewees argued that certain treatments require native language communication, such as child-delivery or psychological counseling. Here, the inequality of access emerges from the near absence of such services. In Germany, for example, there are cases where patients with limited German language skills are purposely excluded from psychological counseling services in hospitals as a psychologist in a hospital notes: "If there is a foreigner, I ask the head-nurse whether he speaks German and if he doesn't I don't go there" (hospital psychologist, gynecological oncology, Bremen, 2006). A further example of unequal access due to language barriers is the limited participation of migrants in delivery room tours conducted in German. In Trento it is difficult for migrants to make an appointment in the hospital because appointments are made by telephone and the procedure is computerized, so there are no people at the other end of the telephone to communicate with. Such a barrier to access is also cited as a challenge for Italians which highlights how difficult this might be for the migrants as noted in the following quote:

> access to services in the health care system is a complex issue also for Italians. When we need to use services we have to get a green number, we have to wait, we have to do this and that, make sure that you are given an appointment after—I do not know—how long of a wait, stamp out a number, press six, press eight … At times it is complicated for us who know how to work the system, who have a manual in their hands. I can imagine what this means for a foreigner who lives here and has very limited knowledge of the system, the language and way to communicate. He or she cannot speak with the secretaries, does not know the procedures … does not understand. But what does it mean not to understand, you have to try over and over again, because there is no one you can ask. From my perspective it is a complex issue. (Migrant Association, Naples, 2007)

In Leipzig it was also noted that patients with articulation problems run the risk of not being understood by the medical staff. "Migrants usually visit doctors, who speak their mother tongue. But if they have a complicated illness, then they go to German doctors. Here comes the point of misunderstanding" (language and culture mediator from Russia, Leipzig, 2007). Service providers in Vancouver also noted that these communication gaps bring up concerns about patient risk and the ability of patients to provide informed consent when misunderstandings are so prevalent. For example it was noted in Vancouver that a parent was unsure of the reason behind her child's surgery because an interpreter was not used to ensure she understood. In Bremen some alluded to similar cases where in the aftermath of an operation migrants would not be informed about the type of and reason for the operation. Also, misunderstanding regarding prescriptions is seen as another significant risk by respondents in Canada and Italy.

Therefore two significant issues surface with respect to how language barriers play out in the system. First, access might be limited due to language skills because migrants do not have the communication skills required in order to effectively navigate the health care system. Second, language barriers may limit access to care due to the communication gap between the medical staff and the patient. Respondents noted that this barrier is not exclusive to migrants, since medical knowledge is not accessible to the native-born population as well. However, migrants are doubly challenged due to both the language skills and the mastery of the medical vocabulary for communicating with the medical staff for their needs.

The lack of interpretation services across the continuum of care was seen as a significant concern in Vancouver: "if they need to go to a specialist, the specialists don't provide interpreters" (program manager, community clinic, Vancouver, 2006), and another respondent stated that: "interpretation services are kind of piecemeal. Some services have some languages and some others don't" (doctor, hospital clinic, Vancouver, 2006). It was also noted that, in Vancouver, interpretation services were only regularly available at the hospital, and not at all in most community health centers. In contrast to this, community health centers in Montreal have more interpreter service usage than is found in the hospital setting.

Migrants' dependence on family members for translation services in f the absence of professional translation services in our case studies from Germany is said to reduce their access to only basic care, while excluding them from special services such as the use of midwives during pregnancy.[5] Inadequate translation efforts of non-professional interpreters and basic comprehension difficulties prevent an adequate registration of the medical history, as well as satisfactory diagnostics.

> If someone comes with a broken leg, I can take an X-ray image. Then I basically tell him that he is not allowed to walk with that leg for five weeks. But if someone comes who has abdominal pain, I have to ask for details. This is an issue which a simple 'Do-you-speak-German?' can't solve. (Medical Director of the University Clinic, Leipzig, 2007)

5 Bremen is one of two federal German states that offers so-called family midwives. These midwives are targeting socially marginalized families. Their service goes beyond the basic midwife service, also addressing child-care issues and access to social service structures.

Since the use of interpreters does not constitute a medical service which is covered by health insurance, translators have to be obtained from elsewhere. While hospitals generally fall back on foreign-speaking staff and, in rare cases, an interpreter service, ambulatory clinics often rely on family members: "An established doctor is not getting more money because he deals with a foreign patient. Therefore, he first asks the patient whether he has someone in the family, who can translate for him" (employee of the advice center for migrants, Leipzig, 2006).

In all three countries health care workers, not the patient, decide if an interpreter or mediator is needed. The majority of translation services in the health sector in Leipzig occur voluntarily and without training. Even in places where there is access to interpretation services, many people noted that interpretation was either not used at all or other staff or family members would be relied upon for interpretation. In Trento the service is underused because many workers are still unaware of the service or prefer to speed up the visit with the patient and therefore proceed without mediators.

In Germany it is not uncommon that children are involved as translators (for example in gynecology): "Yes that is why I say, the children are able to translate much better. They come with their young daughters, are ashamed a little while, it's something embarrassing, but at least they can. It is still in the family" (medical doctor, hospital, Leipzig, 2006). In Canada it was also noted that family members are often used for translation services, although most people spoke of the inappropriateness of using family members for medical interpretation.[6] A migrant association suggested that immigrants themselves need to be made aware of the problems with inappropriate interpretation, and to make the demand: "your 13-year-old kid doesn't have to do the interpretation for you when you're talking to a doctor about sensitive matters; you have the right to an interpreter" (representative, Migrant Association, Vancouver, 2006). Migrant associations noted that inappropriate interpretation practices are common: "people sometimes arrive with their relative or they go to a hospital at emergency and they go to find a janitor for the translation, because he's the only one that speaks the language" (representative, Migrant Association, Montreal, 2006). In Vancouver, service providers also noted problems with interpretation practices: "Some are still using their staff to do interpretations … or using family members to do interpretation which again is inappropriate because some sensitive information might be missed" (doctor, hospital clinic, Vancouver, 2006).

The cost of hiring interpreters is a key aspect in the discourse of migration and health in Germany. While medical staff seldom claim a statutory regulation for any interpretation services, migrant representatives and politicians demand access to translation service for a fee. Proposals regarding a uniform approach to organizing interpretation services have been rejected by the national hospital

6 The use of family members for translation purposes is also a highly contested issue in the German health care system: while some see it as a pragmatic response others are adamantly opposed to this practice.

society in 2007 and the national minister for integration is reluctant to follow up on the issue. Whether there should be a main institution or an interpreter pool is often debated. So far, the city of Leipzig provides an annual budget for a total of 50 single interpreter services, that refugees can call upon. A translator service for legal migrant residents in Leipzig does not exist. In Trento and Naples there is no mediation service organized inside hospitals, as it would cost too much and there are not sufficient resources. In Naples mediation and linguistic services have fewer resources than in Trento. It was noted by community liaison personnel in Montreal that often the choice not to use interpreter services is because of the cost: "It costs institutions money, and so some institutions are not too willing to use this bank. They will use staff members, which don't necessarily guarantee their confidentiality and the quality of the interpretation" (Diversity program manager, Montreal, 2006).

In addition to the cost of interpretation, another barrier to proper communication between the health service provider and the patient is a question of time. In both Italy and Canada it was expressed that in clinics and hospitals, workers are pressed for time and cannot dedicate the necessary time to interact with a patient with linguistic-cultural differences who needs additional time to communicate effectively.

Legal Status of Immigrants and Issues of Access

The legal status of immigrants and refugees creates significant variance among the type of services people are eligible to receive. In Canada all immigrants must wait for three months before they are granted access to public medical insurance, which is identified as a significant barrier for immigrants. It was seen simply as a denial of service access that needs to be addressed. Government-assisted refugees have access to some health care services, and the Interim Federal Health Program provides funding for basic and emergency care. Despite the access that refugees have to the Interim Federal Health Program, a service provider in Vancouver identified a variety of problems with accessing services. For example, under the IFHP this service provider noted that "in order to get the more complex procedures, the doctors have to write a letter, and it takes time, even for a small surgery, and then it takes time for it to be approved" (program manager, community clinic, Vancouver, 2006).

In Germany irregular migrants and asylum-seekers lack the legal framework for full access (Falge et al. 2009). Residence permit and related work permits determine migrants' access to medical insurance. Asylum-seekers fall under the asylum law (Asylbewerberleistungsgesetz, AsylbLG), a law passed in 1993 which for the first time defined asylum-seekers and refugees as groups of foreigners who are not fully entitled to welfare services including health care. The AsylbLG has severely cut down asylum-seekers and refugees' access to services below the level of citizens with legal residence. The majority of migrants are insured with the statutory health insurance. Ethnic Germans from the former Soviet Union have free access to the statutory health insurance up to one and a half years of duration of stay. Migrants with a permanent legal residence permit and regular and high income as well as foreigners with a three-year minimum duration of stay are legally entitled to access to private insurances. Both groups have equal access symbolized by a health insurance card, and pay additional fees for special services, for example dental care, and so on. Asylum-seekers who have been in Germany for less than four years and who mostly have not acquired work permits are only eligible to limited services, and by specific doctors, excluding them from the freedom of choice for medical institutions.[7] Irregular migrants have no legal rights in health care, but in some states are offered limited access either by an informal, voluntary provider network and/or by a formal system that guarantees anonymous services to protect them from deportation. Health care for irregular migrants was mentioned in the Social Democratic–Green Coalition Treaty of 2007 and thereafter implemented by the Bureau of Public Health Bremen which offers weekly anonymous medical consultations for irregular migrants (Lotze 2009). As a result only health care in cases of essential need or acute emergency is guaranteed.

All other services in Germany beyond urgent care entail bureaucratic obstacles for different categories of patients (irregular migrants, asylum-seekers, legal residents). The following quote summarizes the situation in Germany: "In some cases it is not obvious whether a pain or an acute treatment is necessary. In this case the hospitals and asylum applicants have to demand approval by the foreigners' registration office" (Health Department, Leipzig, 2007). What is recognized as an emergency, though, is not necessarily decided by the medical profession. Chronic diseases, which require longer-term therapy, are often not treated. Also, precautionary measures such as vaccinations have been approved for the children of asylum-seekers. Cancer screening is not provided by statute in the medical service package for migrants without a legal residence status. Regarding the legal framework, the scope of medical services for asylum-seekers in Leipzig, as well as in other parts of Saxony, are very narrow and not yet sufficiently regulated: "It must be ensured that in the case of illness, injury or pregnancy the medical care is guaranteed: But that has not been regulated by the legislature yet" (Commissioner for Foreigners, Leipzig, 2007). Again, access depends on locality and the political will of the authorities to provide health access to migrants and or refugees. Bremen for instance finances two permanent doctors who are based in asylum homes and provide regular services to all asylum-seekers. This is not the case in Leipzig where the political will is largely absent.

In Montreal program managers noted that a key issue for refugees was that they often needed services that are not covered and that they could not pay for. This denial of access to services creates an ethical problem for care providers:

---

7 Since 2007 asylum-seekers with a temporary residence permit (Duldung) are included in the statutory health insurance.

> What are essential services, where is family responsibility for a refugee claimant, but they need more than they're allowed, or someone that doesn't have a status or whose status is ambivalent or they're in-between applying and they have to pay and they can't pay. Someone with mental health issues. There are a lot of issues around that. Because physicians and healthcare professionals feel frustrated because they're obliged to give service, ethically, but the systems in place don't always coincide. Here they're working on policies. But it really needs a bigger initiative from the government, and a concerted effort across the board. (Diversity program manager, hospital, Montreal, 2006)

In Leipzig refugees who are in tolerated status but still expect deportation anytime often avoid medical services because they are concerned about their right of residence: "From people without residence status, we have less requests; they have concerns that we are a state authority and that this may trigger intervention by the police or even deportation" (board member of the children and youth advisory board Kaktus e.V., Leipzig, 2007). The legislation in Germany (which is unique in the entire EU) forbids asylum-seekers to leave the district assigned to them by the Department of Immigration. In the case of crossing the compulsory boundaries, asylum-seekers are threatened with a prison sentence of up to one year. Similar concerns exist among refugees or irregular immigrants in Canada. In Vancouver a service provider at an immigrant clinic noted that many people who are in a precarious immigration situation often do not use health services because of their concerns of being deported.

In Italy, in principle, the full inclusion of legal immigrants in the National Health System (NHS) is guaranteed by Act no. 40/98 and by T.U. 286/98 in the articles 34 and 35, but, as we will see, in practice a rich region such as Trentino is able to offer better services to all users, including migrants. According to such norms foreigners regularly present,[8] even if unemployed, are entitled to the same rights as Italian citizens. Compulsory registration with the NHS is guaranteed during the validity of the residence permit, in order to achieve stability for the whole duration of the residence period and its continuity is guaranteed during the time needed for permit renewal. The enrolment ends only in cases of non-renewal or repeal of the residence permit, or in case of expulsion. Health care is also extended to the family dependents regularly living together,[9] and the registration

8 This means legally resident foreigners who have regular dependent jobs or are self-employed or are registered in the job center's lists; legally resident foreigners who have asked for the renewal of the residence permit for work reasons, for self-employment, family reasons, political refugees, humanitarian asylum-seekers requesting asylum, for adoption, for foster care, for citizenship application. Those who do not fit into these categories, and have a residence permit for more than three months, must sign an insurance policy against the risk of illness, accidents and also in case of maternity with an Italian or foreign insurance company. One can also enroll in the NHS on a voluntary basis, paying a yearly contribution.

9 Previously the family dependents had the possibility of enrolling only on a voluntary basis and therefore had to pay a yearly fee.

in the NHS is guaranteed from birth to children of foreigners registered with the NHS. The enrolment is carried out at the local health unit where one has residence.

In order to safeguard individual and collective health, health care services are, however, also guaranteed to people without private insurance or voluntary registration with the NHS. The case of irregular migrants, foreigners who—although legally entitled to registration—do not appear on record, and foreigners who entered the country for tourism or business reasons, are expected to pay for the treatment if they hold a private insurance policy. The NHS ensures that irregular foreigners are entitled to urgent, continuing and essential outpatient and hospital care[10] and all the health care necessary to prevent illness or accidents. The inclusion in the NHS of the irregular immigrants has been organized by regions autonomously, each choosing its own solutions. In some regions, such as Campania, irregular migrants are admitted in "dedicated" outpatient surgeries. In other regions, such as Trentino, irregular migrants are granted free access to general practitioners and pediatric physicians, for the prescription of medicines or specialist clinics.

Irregular immigrants are assigned an anonymous regional ID code (SPT: Straniero Temporaneamente Presente—temporary present immigrant), which is valid for six months and allows the immigrant to use health care services in the same manner as Italians. Article 35 of the T.U. 286/98 also points out that access to the health care system by an immigrant must not be reported to police authorities, except when it is compulsory (for instance reporting is mandatory when a crime may have occurred). Irregular immigrants are assured basic services such as pregnancy and maternity services, the protection of minors' health, diagnosis and care of contagious diseases and prevention, treatment and rehabilitation of toxic dependencies, according to the rules and within the areas of intervention set by the regions. In the case of irregular migrants, no payment for treatment is required "if they are without the necessary economic resources, excluding the payment of the charges as Italian citizens have to pay." In order to enjoy these rights, immigrants have to fill in an official form declaring that they lack sufficient economic resources (Dichiarazione di Indigenza), and the Minister of Interiors refunds the expenses incurred. Even if there is no discernible difference regarding envisaged rights for legal immigrants, there is a significant variation in terms of the capacity to enjoy these rights. On the issue of access to health care services, it depends mainly on the personal commitment of social and medical workers encountered while the services are being received. There are people in the system

10 A memorandum of the Health Ministry, n.5 of March 24, 2000, Indicazioni applicative del decreto legislativo 25 luglio 1998, n. 286 defined urgent treatments as those that cannot be deferred without putting life at risk or damaging people's health; and essential treatments as diagnostic and therapeutic interventions for pathologies not immediately dangerous, but that over time could provoke a damage to health or risks for life, due to complications, chronically or worsening.

who are more open-minded and willing to facilitate access, with particularly good examples in the field of maternity care.

In recent years a set of new regulations have qualified in more restrictive terms the norms in the Law 286 of 1998 concerning immigration, and specifically the relation between immigration and health. There are more restrictive norms concerning residence requirements to access health services. Also migrants often face limitations due to health standards as restricting factors in other policy sectors. For instance there are currently new and generally more stringent health standards required in obtaining housing permits, which hinder migrants who out of necessity often seek to live in substandard housing. These changes are on the one hand meant to protect public health but on the other hand make access more difficult for migrants. However, in some cases there have also been enabling opportunities. For instance, migrants can currently extend their residence permit in case it should expire when the migrant is ill or had an occupational accident that hinders departure. In general, the legal situation of migrants and refugees is becoming more restricted since the political turn to the right that has characterized Italy in recent years. The exception is the few instances in which more tolerant laws are approved as they originate at the European level, such as two anti-racist directives connected to the approval of article 13 of the Amsterdam Treaty.

In the 1990s, politicians and civil society organizations in Italy agreed that looking after irregular immigrants' health is important to protect the health of everybody. The link between the status of the immigrant and his/her access to health care services is a highly politicized issue that permeates into public opinion as anti-immigration rhetoric. This is because of the widely held belief that immigrants are a burden to the social system and do not contribute to making the system sustainable (the so-called welfare chauvinism) and the public fear that immigrants are the carriers of illnesses (the so-called Salgari Syndrome[11]).

In particular, in recent times, the spread of fears and alarmist ideas from certain political actors reflecting a criminalization and securitization of immigrants has led to questioning the already accomplished rights of immigrants. In 2009 the government played with the idea that doctors be required to report irregular immigrants when they access services in the health care system. Already many immigrants have not used these services often, partly because they are afraid to trust doctors given limited or misguided information on this issue. Now there is all the more reason for irregular immigrants not to use the structures of the health care system. Migrants' irregularity is widely perceived to be of extremely high proportion in Italy and these laws can only have a hindering impact on their willingness to use the health services.[12]

11 The name "Salgari syndrome" originates from the Italian novelist who, though never travelling out of Italy, perfectly described environments and habits typical of distanced countries. The term warns of such stereotypes.

12 For opinion data on the relevance of irregular migration in Italy see the international research project "Transatlantic Trends 2010," www.gmfus.org/trends/2010/index.html.

In Canada the health services for migrants and refugees are also uncertain in terms of their availability and quality. Respondents in Montreal have noticed the deterioration over time in the services available for refugees and migrants: "there are periods when it's a little better, and periods when it's worse. Now they're not offering very much" (Diversity program manager, hospital, Montreal, 2006). And another program manager noted that "being an immigrant in Canada ten years ago was easier than being an immigrant in Canada today" (Diversity program manager, hospital, Montreal, 2006).

Economic Issues: The Restraints on the System and Migrants

Economic conditions create a problem for access to care, both because of the precarious personal economic situation that many immigrants are in, and due to the economic restraints in health care spending generally, and specifically the limited financing of programs targeted to minorities, including funding for associations. In Canada, shortages of resources and personnel in the health care setting have led to a decline in the coverage of services for refugees, and a deterioration in services received for immigrants in Montreal over the past few years. Immigrants and program managers in Montreal noted that the changes in the health care system have created more access barriers, with fewer health workers available in areas such as maternity care: "some of them will say that before, when my first child was born … I had more, I was able to access more easily than when my third child was born. Because more health workers were available" (midwife, community clinic, Montreal, 2006). In Vancouver it was also noted that limited resources for health practitioners and service provision were identified. In a clinic for immigrants the staff expressed this concern:

> We have limited resources, very limited resources. For example, I have part-time here, even though I could be working full-time, but there is no money for us. Even for the doctors, 'cause we are crowded, we have lots of people here. And we don't have—we are only open from 1:00–4:00 Monday to Friday. And some specialized clinics, like chronic illnesses, children, you know pediatric clinic—but we don't have money to be open like for a full day. (Program manager, community clinic, Vancouver, 2006)

Economic restraint is a significant issue for Italian health care, but it's more about services not being offered or underutilized rather than services being cut (for instance less use of mediation services). Such discrepancy is noted in the following quote:

> And hence for people gravely sick, those who need urgent care for instance during their pregnancy or because of an accident, we have public institutions that are very open and strictly obligated to attend to these people in need. To

> me this seems to be a positive characteristic from the viewpoint of solidarity. (Expert/professor, Milan, 2008)

Regional economic variation creates a situation where the poorer communities, where many immigrants live, have poorer services available. The political will to launch specific programs such as mediation services, dedicated ambulatory, training for workers, prevention campaigns and so on, are simply not there in several German states. In Canada it was also noted that dedicated health services for immigrants are not seen as part of the core mandate of the public health care system, and therefore are not prioritized for funding. In Vancouver and Montreal migrant associations noted that funding resources were decreasing, and they have been forced to compete with each other for the shrinking resources for immigrant services project funding, and an ongoing lack of certainty regarding funding.

In all three countries it was also noted that immigrants usually are working in jobs that do not allow them the flexibility for making medical appointments. Work schedules limit the utilization of general practitioners, so a lot of people use emergency care for non-urgent problems. In this section we focus on the economic and financial constraints in the health care system and how this interacts with the socio-economic status of the migrants. The increase in poverty in Canada overall was also seen as contributing to ongoing access barriers for immigrants:

> when you don't work or when you are in an uncertain situation, this generates a series of problems in you that belong to recent immigration. But now, the conditions that we used to associate to recent immigration have a tendency to stretch out in time … And since their economic status is precarious, recent immigrants feel very uncomfortable to go take language classes when they should be working. (Program manager, hospital, Montreal, 2006)

In connection with the health care of migrants and their socio-economic status, the educational level of migrants is important. In Germany it was noted that these differences affect access: "I think people coming from the academic sector, or the ones which have been staying here for a longer time, have better access to health care and also demand these benefits more often" (board member of the children and youth advisory board Kaktus e.V., Leipzig, 2007). Migrants' socio-economic status, including their educational level, affects health access. While the rate of student migrants has increased, the unemployment rate of migrants in Saxony is at 41.9 percent and in Bremen at 27.4 percent. Particularly precarious is the economic situation of refugees.

In all three countries it was noted that many immigrants experience downward social mobility. The credentials and work experience of immigrants is often unrecognized, so many people with higher education are not able to find work in their area. A case in point is that most foreign trained doctors who received their degrees in the home country are unable to practice medicine in the receiving country.

In Germany there are also inequalities between privately and statutorily insured patients, with privately insured patients receiving more access privileges and being prioritized over statutorily insured patients: "It matters where you come from and which insurance you have, whether your health costs are covered by the social service or whether you are educated" (hospital nurse, Arabic-speaking, Bremen, 2007). It is also noted that there are growing inequalities between German migrants and a growing number of non-insured Eastern European labor migrants living in Germany without health insurance coverage due to economic reasons.

Lack of Data on the Diversity of the Population

One of the significant barriers in providing appropriate health services to immigrants and refugees in all three countries is that there is inadequate data about communities and their economic situations, about service use and the appropriateness of the services offered, or whether the programs offered specifically for immigrants are successful. For instance in Trento it is not known if the utilization of general practitioners is a successful strategy: local health offices do not differentiate among "tourists," "legal" and "irregular immigrants" so we can't know how many immigrants are using the service. There is some local level data about service utilization and disease profiles, but there is very little available at the national level.

In Canada there is no data on ethnicity or immigration status collected when people use services, so it is impossible to measure if the services are being used by the many communities they are meant to serve. In Vancouver it was noted that there is not adequate data collected to assist in planning:

> because we don't collect ethno-cultural data ... it's very ... idiosyncratic. Like we'll talk to staff and they'll say 'wow, we're seeing huge numbers of people from Eastern Europe' ... We can track ... by looking at census data but, you know we're always a year behind with that. So, we see that there are newer groups that we're starting to serve in different communities within our region, but we don't have a systematic way of capturing the data and then planning a response that's appropriate. (Program manager, Vancouver, 2006)

At the same time, migrant associations noted that often the issues of concern for migrants were not integrated into planning. For example, in Montreal a strategy for mental health was developed without input from or discussion about minorities and their particular issues in mental health. In general it is seen that the diversity of the population is not taken into account in health care planning.

Interviewees in Leipzig criticized repeatedly that political representatives argue against an extension of the supply of health services for immigrants because of the comparatively low proportion of migrants. "They act purely formal: Is the specialist care secured? Is there an over-supply or a supply disruption? And then they always say: 'Leipzig has supply surplus. Rejected'" (Director of the Health Office, Leipzig, 2007). Yet the ability to assess these figures remains unsolved. "A handicap in this regulation is the lack of statistical data. That no one has reliable figures to say there are so and so many thousands or more" (Commissioner for Foreigners, city of Leipzig, 2007). Therefore the need of action for migrant populations is undermined by the inadequate statistical coverage which means that the problems of migrants are not identified and analyzed. The interviews show that in the health sector in Leipzig, migrants' special needs are only slowly being recognized by the public and medical sphere.

In Germany some official statistics can be used for analyzing the health situation of migrants. These are specific data on social and health coverage, representative studies and surveys (Mikrozensus, Socioeconomic Panel, and so on). These data sources provide representative and frequently collected data on aspects of health and include more or less information about the migrant background of the participants. Most of these data sources allow the identification of migrants based on nationality. However, definition of migrants based on nationality will exclude the majority of persons with migrant background in Germany, who are naturalized migrants or ethnic German migrants with German nationality (Razum and Spallek 2006). Only some of the databases include information about previous nationality, nationality of parents, country of origin, the parents' country of origin, or language spoken at home, and so on. An effective health monitoring for migrants does not exist in Germany yet and as a result statistical data on migrants' access to the health system and about how the system is used by migrants in Germany is not available. How big the additional expenses are for the medical profession when they treat migrants is seen differently: while resident doctors tend to speak about a small percentage of treated migrants, counseling centers speak in that context of such an extensive effort, they claim that their professional, personal and financial capacity is not sufficient.

> We are in the process of building a contact point where foreign patients can go to and articulate certain claims or suggestions for improvement. Then we are going to sort out the data: who is this patient? What kind of needs does this person lack? Which language does this person speak? So that they are guided from A to Z. (Member, hospital medical board, Leipzig, 2006)

What counts as a specific need remains mostly vague or unclear due to differing views between the various players and decision-making bodies: "Between the doctors and the public health service there are often arguments and different opinions about what a patient needs in the standard health supply and what not" (Director of the Health Office, Leipzig, 2007). Reflecting the particularities of the local context in Leipzig there is a lack of networking between medical staff and migrant associations that are able to articulate the needs of migrants. Concrete elaborated concepts, which take needs of migrants into account, exist only marginally. The lack of direct communication is repeatedly criticized: "For example Gekomm is a very good thing. Prevention must be more elaborate than the treatment … But what I think is sometimes missing is a little more contact between the involved and participating actors" (cultural and linguistic mediator, Leipzig, 2008).

Apart from these general points, a quantification of the general situation of access and types of usage of the health system is limited by the paucity and limited scope of data. Information on migrants' access and utilization of the Italian health system is still collected in a partial and unsystematic manner. However, some examples will suffice to describe the main features of immigrants' usage. At the local level there are a number of research projects on issues of migrants' access, but they are not sufficiently coordinated among the various regions and it is difficult to form a convincing picture of the situation at the national level. Available data at the national level concern hospital and day-hospital discharge reports but no recent data are available. On the basis of available data it is possible to draw some conclusions even if they are limited by insufficient regional coverage, distortions and difficulty in the analysis over time. For example, it is not possible to differentiate between legal and irregular immigrant patients. However, the existing data show that the services to foreign patients have increased over time. The existing data also suggest a different type of usage by migrant patients. For instance, for females there is a much higher request for fertility care and abortion services. For males, there is a high incidence of hospital admission for traumas and other work-related issues, and problems with the digestive system. The previously high level of infectious illnesses seems to have decreased in recent years, whilst the number of work-related incidents remains very high—143,651 work-related accidents in 2009, 176 of them resulting in death (see Caritas Italiana—Fondazione Migrantes 2010).

Although in all our cases, some health-related data of people with an immigrant background are collected, there is no standardized way of compiling these data and, as a result, it is hard to make comparisons. Against this background it is difficult to create homogenous and comparable clinical files, as also noted by the following quote: "Since this information is not available it becomes impossible to compare these clinical files … Over the past ten years there has not been a monitoring system in place for hospitals" (expert/professor, Milan, 2008).

As already mentioned, effective health monitoring for migrants and migrant-specific statistical data in the health sector are absent in Germany. Similarly, neither hospitals nor general practitioners collect these data which makes it difficult to determine migrants' level of access to the health care system and to develop migrant-friendly health care services.

Conclusions

To conclude this discussion of access, it is important to point out that levels of access are constantly changing for a variety of factors, some external to the efforts of any social and political actor, others emerging from coordinated efforts. Civil society groups obtain, re-negotiate and where possible expand access via an interplay of strategies and the institutional structures. Historical developments, such as changes in public opinion on multiculturalism and variations in the number of migrants, also play a role in expanding and restricting access.

Therefore the differential access and use of services may be attributed to many reasons. The level of system or institutional supports to enhance access (adequate translation, inter-cultural training, migrant-specific programs) shape migrants' experiences with health care services. In addition, barriers to access may originate from the characteristics of those who try to access the system, with variation within and between ethnic groups demonstrating that access is multi-dimensional, with differences between urban and rural, across neighborhoods, and between the genders. Class, ethnicity and gender reinforce each other in both marginalizing groups themselves and restricting access to the health care system due to these group characteristics.

This chapter presented the ways in which, despite general commitments to provision of equal treatment in health care to all, the different countries reveal variation in practice. Such differences in practice are observed in the barriers around service knowledge, different uses of the health care services, the geographical location of the migrant, different access level across sectors in the health care system, differences arising from cultural diversity or legal status, language barriers, economic matters pertaining to the system and individuals, and the lack of data on people with migrant backgrounds accessing the system. The barriers suggest that in all cases the attitudes toward providing equal treatment in principle are less often realized in practice, as barriers to equality exist, and equal treatment may not be adequate to meet the migrants' needs that may be exacerbated by ethnicity, class and gender differences. The barriers discussed here identify points of stress in the health care system as it aims to address challenges arising from diversity. A significant issue that arises is the way in which local cultures impact the ways and means through which migrants' needs are addressed in the system.

The chapter discusses the findings for the cases of Canada, Germany and Italy on the barriers to access to the health system. The findings indicate that the main barriers to equitable and culturally-sensitive services originate from how the health care system is institutionalized, how the service providers practice their work, and the extent to which the immigrants are equipped to operate within the health care systems of the receiving countries. Observing the various difficulties, a few concluding remarks are in order. First, the findings indicate that the barriers to access have multiple origins and hence require action at multiple levels with coordinated action among multiple stakeholders. For example the health care systems themselves have financial problems, questions of funding priorities (language services vs. another operation room) and unequal delivery of services (regional variation, privately vs. statutorily insured patients in Germany), which require attention for immigrants and non-immigrants alike to improve the services.

Second, the systems do include an acknowledgment of the needs of diversity at least in legislation. However, when it comes to implementing such principles by prioritizing diversity-based needs, all the systems fall short of realizing the ideal. Third, there are organized efforts to overcome barriers by collective action of migrants through associations, yet the link between the mobilization or political advocacy of migrants and improved access is impacted by various structural, agency and cultural factors. Some of the structural factors relate to how the systems within the different cases organize migrants' participation in the formulation of health care policy and practice. Another issue stems from whether migrants have their own leading individuals or groups who will champion the need to overcome barriers in the health care system. Another matter relates to how different migrant or minority groups operate in the different cases with or without the mediation of associations. The strategies in the system as a whole to overcome these challenges will be explored in the next chapter.

Chapter 5
Strategies for Change among Institutional and Civil Society Actors

Saime Ozcurumez and Lloy Wylie

This chapter will first provide background on the political and regulatory frameworks of Germany, Canada and Italy, as this is the legislation that qualifies access to health services. This allows us to highlight how the essential regulatory frameworks are both a considerable constraint and opportunity for civil society and migrant organizations. They also allow us to show the dynamic nature of the relation between state and civil society—more specifically, between state and organized civil society. In each of the countries we consider, civil society develops in ways that are in part isomorphic and in part complementary to the structure of the state. Each of the states we examine support civil society in different ways and for different purposes, and in doing so shape the way pro-migrant associations operate. The first section of this chapter will illustrate these processes. We will then move to examine how civil society actors have become engaged in the field of health care and what strategies they have adopted in our national contexts. Finally, we will examine what policy lessons can be learned from our case studies, both in terms of access and in terms of policy effectiveness in the service delivery and advocacy functions.

The Regulatory and Institutional Framework: Policy-Making in Health Care

The legal and regulatory framework for governing health care differs substantially in the three national contexts. This is of critical significance for what political strategies are developed in order to bring about institutional changes in how health care systems accommodate diversity. Who has the primary responsibility for the development and implementation of services, at what level of government are these procedures negotiated and what are the appropriate channels to gain "voice" in the decision-making process? As we will discuss in the first section of this chapter, there are a host of contextual factors that shape the scope and format of political advocacy in Canada, Germany and Italy. Some are directly related to the legal-regulatory framework within which the health care system operates. Others are more related to the broader political opportunities and constraints that result from modes of governance and division of policy competences across territorial levels or the dynamic of competitive party politics.

The Political and Regulatory Framework in Germany

As already mentioned in preceding chapters, the attitude of politicians and program managers in Bremen toward migrant-specific care is mainly framed by a universalist approach. Though the 'integration guidelines' in Bremen specifically recommend the intercultural aperture of health services, the integration officer argued in an interview with us that the universalist health care system makes the intercultural aperture unnecessary (administrative state representative for integration, Bremen, 2005). Hence, it is hardly surprising to find that legal enforcements in terms of an intercultural opening[1] (ICO) are almost non-existent in the German context. Part of the reason for the lack of ICO may be attributed to the extent that political change is reflected in hospital settings, which is observable in the ways in which the political system, the health care system and hospital management interact with each other.

In 2003, Bremen's four public hospitals were merged under a larger structure called "Klinikum Nord." While formerly the communes were represented in the technical supervision of health care provision ("*Fachaufsicht*"), policy-makers are now represented in the respective governing board ("*Aufsichtsrat*") of the hospitals. With this arrangement, the regional government has virtually lost its political influence in the hospital (particularly the legal framework defining its *modus operandi*) and is solely involved in the hospital planning committee, which focuses on management questions such as budget cuts, reductions in the number of beds and mergers of departments. Therefore, instead of a legal obligation to abide by a larger ICO framework, initiatives depend on the clinic director and the interest, motivation and commitment of personnel. As a result, the level of ICO therefore differs among the various hospitals.

Despite a decentralized structure of political intervention, the senator of health oversees the provision of health care. The Bremen Bureau of Public Health (BoH) emphasizes the participation of all citizens, particularly those considered as socially marginalized, in initiatives for health promotion, including ICO. The Bremen BoH is widely known for its progressiveness and pro-migrant attitude. The office is mandated to create healthy living conditions, protect individuals and groups from negative health effects, strengthen self-responsibility and provide necessary health support (BoH 2000: 5). Cooperation with other partners working in the area of health care is encouraged and should take place through responsible guidance and equal partnership. In 1993, the BoH in Bremen established the

1 We define intercultural opening in terms of intercultural training programs offered to hospital staff, number of immigrants employed in all levels of the hospital hierarchy, translation services, multi-linguistic information materials, multi-linguistic sign boards, multi-religious facilities and food, visitors rooms, etc.

Department for Migration and Health, which focuses on asylum seekers, refugees and ethnic Germans' reception centers.

The majority of migrants and non-migrants in Germany are insured with the statutory health insurance according to the social health insurance code (SGB V), which also covers family members. Ethnic Germans from the former Soviet Union have free access to the statutory health insurance up to one and a half years of duration of stay. Three of the four employees of the Department of Migration and Health (the head and two general practitioners) have a migration background. The Department provides health care for refugees and asylum seekers and has developed concepts for migrant-specific elderly care and a multilingual guide about insurance for welfare recipients (*Pflegeversicherung*). It has also established a pool of translators (*Dolmetscherpool*) and produced a health-guide-post (*Gesundheitswegweiser*), which provides information on the language skills of general practitioners and medical specialists. The head of the BoH was also a key actor in establishing Refugio, the trauma center for refugees. Other organizations working in the area of ICO reported great difficulties in matters of cooperation with the BoH, as it was seen as dominating the field of migrant health and reluctant to cooperate with other actors.[2]

Quality control is one method through which legal norms concerning ICO are enforced in the health care sector in Germany. Hospitals in Germany are part of a quality certification system which measures quality of service provided along set and common standards. Despite the fact that intercultural training has not become a part of quality certification, since 2005 all hospitals in Bremen and most technical training programs (*Fachausbildungen*) have started to offer ICO courses, for which demand is steadily increasing.[3] Those trainees that have been through the ICO programs argue that their working conditions are decisively improving due to their acquired intercultural skills (although this training is not mandatory).

Introducing Services for Migrants: The Role of Civil Society Actors in Germany

The AWO (*Workers Welfare Organization*) is one of the six leading welfare work associations in Germany. At the European Union (EU) level, it is a member of the EU-based organization SOLIDAR, which promotes workers' rights with a special program for migrant domestic workers. Since the early 1960s, the AWO-Bremen has provided services for migrants including a special department for migration. While initially services were only offered to immigrants, in the early

2 The BoH Leipzig does not consider migrants' health care access in similar ways as the Bremen office. They nevertheless prepared a health guide similar to the one in Bremen. Both health guides are however hardly used by migrants.

3 These training courses are offered by a XENOS project called "Health Intercultural." Prior to the XENOS project's establishment in 2005, the project's trainer had offered courses on a private basis. Nursing schools actually integrated ICO courses in their curricula, though for fewer credits than other courses.

1990s the institution also began to address the needs of refugees and asylum seekers. The AWO-Bremen has continually adjusted its services to the steady growth of the number of migrants in Germany. Currently, the AWO-Bremen supports the integration of immigrants by promoting participation in all areas of social, cultural and political life. Since 2005, the tasks have been adjusted to the new immigration law.

The AWO has taken over the first Counseling of Migrants (MEB) and the Youth Migration Services (JMD). The MEB provides support for the integration of immigrants. The AWO has also been adjusting their institutions to the concept of ICO. In total, 10 percent of the AWO-Bremen's employees are migrants. The Department of Migration addresses health issues by participating in the nationwide campaign for culturally sensitive nursing, as well as by offering intercultural training courses. The Department of Migration frequently receives requests for mediation from the hospitals, as it is well known that many of its staff are immigrants. Hence, several institutions in Bremen that encounter communication / translation problems with Turkish migrants refer those cases to the AWO migration department. Due to the inadequacy of translation services in hospitals the Turkish employee of the department is also called in to assist in issues involving patients of Turkish origin—several times in the context of suicide attempts.

Another key initiative to improve access for migrants comes from institutions focusing on a particular area of health care provision. One prominent example from Bremen is the Institute for Psycho-social Work and Prevention for Migrants (DEVA). DEVA is one of three non-governmental institutions in Bremen that employs psychologists and psychotherapists with a migration background. Founded in 1986 as an umbrella organization for female therapists, DEVA initially offered sport and relaxation programs for mixed German/Turkish women's groups. As of 1989, it began to exclusively focus on immigrants (adults and children), and has conducted a needs assessment on the psychosocial needs of immigrants. In 2001, DEVA was officially recognized as an agency for 'child and youth affairs' and received contracts to provide youth services.[4]

There are two other civil society organizations that provide services to the most vulnerable among the migrant population. The first is Home Instruction for Parents of Preschool Children (HIPPY), a program which has a main clientele of immigrants. Their primary task is to support families in preparing their children for school, but they also create awareness for psychological illness and connect clients with the mental-health system. The second organization is Refugio, one of the first psychosocial centers in north-west Germany, founded in 1989. Refugio provides psychosocial support to war-traumatized refugees and asylum-seekers, as this group has no legal access to the German health system. Refugio[5] permanently

4 In 2006 government funding for this organization was terminated and the organizations' activities were reduced to a minimum.

5 These figures apply to the time frame of data collection (2005–2008) and might have changed since.

employs one psychotherapist and a political scientist with a migration background. It also employs five part-time psychotherapists, an art therapist, a body therapist, 25 translators and 12 volunteer therapists. Refugio has a very good reputation in Bremen and many prominent actors on its board, such as members from the BoH (head of the migration desk) and Bremen University's Department of Cultural Studies. Refugio also exists in various other German cities and is sponsored by the EU, as well as by private donations.

Similar services in psychosocial care are also developed directly by smaller migrant organizations: The EU-funded project "*Familie im Hilfenetz*" offers psychosocial support to physically challenged immigrants.[6] Another project is *Komijin*, a Kurdish women's association formed in 1989 as an exchange forum, which also offers German classes, leisure activities and counseling. During the weekly consultation hours at the headquarters of the association, many women express physical problems which hint at psychosomatic diseases. The women do, however, strongly object to consulting psychological services due to the stigmatization of mental diseases among the Kurdish/Turkish community. According to a Turkish psychologist invited by the association to brief its members on mental health issues, for instance, the women did not show much interest in information about mental health issues. As these examples point out, the services developed by civil society sector organizations mostly target highly marginalized groups that have no or very limited access to health care services. In terms of the scope and orientation of these services, it is noteworthy that they are developed outside of and complementary to the health care system, rather than provided as incentives for its institutional reform.

Practitioners and Professionals in the Health Care System

Most hospital staff interviewed in Bremen are in favor of migrant-specific services. They promote these services for two reasons: (1) they consider them as a way to lower the access barriers to health care that migrants face; and (2) they view them as economically advantageous for hospitals in a competitive market for health care. Specifically, staff with a migration background strongly encourage the establishment of migrant-friendly services, such as patient self-help groups in psychiatric settings and multilingual guided tours in delivery wards. Many hospitals have organized multilingual information material for migrants, as reported by a social worker from a hospital situated in a migrant-dense city district: "If we have a patient diagnosed with cancer who does not understand the diagnosis, we hand out information material in Turkish" (hospital social worker, Bremen 2007). Staff emphasize the specific importance of migrant-friendly services and care in the post-admission phase: "Especially when patients with a migration background are released, it is important to assure care by institutions

6 Funding for this project was also terminated in 2007 and the association closed down.

with staff with foreign language skills and cultural competence" (hospital social worker, psychiatric ward, Bremen 2007). In Bremen, Russian- and Turkish-speaking ambulatory care services have been established and are recommended for patients with these backgrounds. The few existing migrant-friendly services are often known to migrants: "When it comes to the Turkish-speaking counseling service in town, they know it—it is nothing new to them if we tell them" (social hospital worker, Bremen 2007).

Between social workers there exists opposing narratives with respect to the provision of health care services that pay particular attention to the needs arising from diversity. While staff with a migration background emphasize the need for various migrant-specific care services (such as foreign language-based counseling services in the hospitals' social service sections), German staff argue that migrants do not need these services. Migrant staff argue in favor of such services because they are aware that migrants often have little knowledge about existing health support structures. A three year project that employed a social worker with a migration background in a migrant-dense city district improved migrants' knowledge about and access to social services in the hospital: "This project developed a culture that problems of migrants were more readily recognized and that migrants had a higher willingness to access existing offers, to access counseling rather than remaining defensive" (social worker, Bremen 2007). Non-migrant hospital social workers, on the other hand, argued that migrants are not accessing social services due to their preference to rely on extended family networks.

Some staff with a migration background maintain contact with mosques to help Muslim patients in need of spiritual guidance during mourning and death. Migrant staff are also better informed about migrant-friendly services in the city as a whole. In one of the hospitals, for instance, it was mainly migrant staff that had knowledge about the Muslim prayer room in the hospital's entrance hall and the Russian-speaking self-help group in another hospital. Often it is migrants or their relatives who engage in the improvement of migrant-friendly structures. In one hospital, Muslim staff offered workshops about Islam to create tolerance and understanding for Muslim colleagues and patients.

In Germany the focus is mostly on employing members of migrant communities in the health care system. Hiring migrant staff is considered as one of the central strategies to improve migrants' access to health care by practitioners in Bremen. As a result, hospitals in migrant dense districts started to employ migrants in key positions: "We have a Turkish ward director … and I am sure that he was not chosen without a second thought, because we have a lot of Turkish patients" (hospital nurse, Bremen 2006). The hospital staff usually pointed at migrant colleagues (gynecologists and midwives) to emphasize that their migrant patients had good access to care: "A lot of migrants work in the wards, I would say for Turkish-speaking patients it is usually no problem to find staff that speaks their language" (hospital social worker, Bremen 2006). Internal translation services organized a list indicating the staffs' background of migration and language skills as a strategy to improve access. Besides, all practitioners interviewed in Bremen mentioned their efforts to increase the number of migrant staff: "We have Turkish colleagues on our ward. Of course she is not always on duty, but we also try to employ nurses who know the language" (hospital gynecologist, Bremen, 2006).

Most staff with a migration background nevertheless describe employment in metaphors of struggles. They specifically report about encountering racism and a general lack of funding for migrant-specific services during their struggle for the recognition of their foreign degrees: "It was a fight, a fight and a fight. And now I have a permanent position here in the psychiatric service. And I am the only [Russian] for Bremen" (Russian-speaking psychological counselor, Bremen 2006). New positions are rarely specifically designed for migrant staff, although an exception was for an Iranian psychologist working in Refugio—the trauma center for refugees in Bremen.

Opposing perceptions exist about the significance of language barriers. Non-migrant staff put less emphasis on language barriers while migrant staff specifically address language barriers as a severe constraint for health care access: "there are so many Turkish, Kurdish and Persian speaking women here who face severe language problems" (midwife, Bremen, 2007). Migrant midwives argue that the level of compliance solely depends on their patients' level of understanding and that this is often hampered due to language barriers.

Generally, practitioners in Leipzig expressed a positive attitude toward increasing migrant staff in the health care system. Although they recognize the low ratio of hospital staff from minority cultural backgrounds and the need to increase their numbers, the hospital staff note that due to financial reasons they are against affirmative action: "If I have two equally qualified employees and one is able to speak three more languages, then this of course is an argument for this person. But there is no major argument for affirmative action" (member, Medical Board of the University Hospital, Leipzig, 2006). Alternatively they suggest employing students with a migration background with foreign language skills as translators, especially in university clinics. Some also suggest the establishment of a migrant-specific clinic comprised of migrant staff. The advantages of the model outweighed its disadvantages since on the one hand it would guarantee "optimal health care and one does not need translators as well." While on the other hand it would limit migrant patients from freely deciding a doctor, limiting them to doctors from cultural communities: "patients … would not have a free choice of deciding which doctor they prefer (…) this is in fact a question of legal regulation" (specialist for gynecology and obstetrics, Leipzig, 2006).

Bremen's tradition as a port city has shaped hospitals' encounters with migrants and hence the city is familiar with the need for translation services. In the face of an increasing permanent migrant population however some health training centers have started to target migrant trainees. The midwifery training centers near Bremen train migrant midwives with foreign degrees and promote their acceptance in Bremen hospitals. Just as in Leipzig however, few program managers favored affirmative action by arguing that quality of caregiver should not be determined by a person's migrant background.

Some program managers in Bremen, specifically those working in institutions with a high density of migrant clients, argue that migrant staff facilitates efficient care for migrant patients. The foreigners' department has therefore established affirmative action and one of the welfare institutions exclusively employs migrants for its migrants' help desk section. When it comes to the health care system, a nursing director remarked that members from the second generation of former 'guest workers' have qualified as a generation of fresh graduates who are in the process of taking up employment in health care, specifically in the hospitals' birth wards as midwives. Similar to arguments by doctors and nurses mentioned above, program directors frequently emphasize migrants in key positions as a pull factor to attract migrant patients: "such a head physician, who specifically cares for that type of patients, attracts very different kind of patients" (hospital nursing director, Bremen, 2007).

Affirmative action is generally rejected by policy-makers and practitioners in Leipzig considering it as 'unequal treatment'. A recommended strategy by Leipzig policy-makers is to increase the ratio of staff with a migration background in German institutions which promotes the granting of work permits for foreign students with medical degrees. Furthermore, they argue in favor of mixed work teams. Migrant medical staff are encouraged to function as mediators in society at large, not just in migrant-associations but also in universities, nursing homes, clinics and health offices that policy-makers and practitioners can rely on.

In interviews with Leipzig policy-makers and practitioners, they expressed their approval for increasing the migrant ratio among the working population, specifically to improve communication. These politicians however clearly discourage the employment of migrants in political institutions arguing that this would contradict the German institutional culture: "If people call us in a foreign language we answer to these calls but we will not employ people with foreign language skills to serve those calls" (health policy expert, Leipzig 2007). Interestingly enough, in Leipzig translation services are not necessarily considered as part of institutional responsibility. Some politicians even view it as the partial responsibility of the patient:

> This allowance for special expenditure is perceived ambivalently by different bodies: Nevertheless it must be restricted or controlled with questionnaires and should be paid by the concerned patients. Surely the offer must be enforced but it should not be recognized as part of the general services. (Health policy expert, Leipzig, 2007)

Hospitals in all German cities usually declare Muslim food as vegetarian and have no facilities to prepare other meals. In Bremen, however, they do allow migrants' relatives to bring food. What actually is a transfer of responsibility to provide meals to the patient is defined by hospital staff as part of the cultural aperture. Furthermore, interviewees from Bremen mentioned the following migrant-friendly services which exist in the city: Muslim prayer and visitors rooms; multilingual flyers; nationality-based guided delivery ward tours; overnight family rooms; internal translation pools; multilingual sign boards; high levels of tolerance toward large family attendance in delivery wards; cultural mediators; contacts with religious leaders in the context of death, mourning and funerals; contacts with psychologists with a migration background; women's groups about "traditional" childbed rituals; an Ethics Commission with a branch for migrant concerns; and publications about migration and women's health. These services are far more limited in Leipzig.[7]

When asked for strategies that could improve migrants' health care access, interviewees from Bremen mentioned: migrant-based self-help groups (so far hardly existent); call-on-help structures; awareness training about rights in care organizations; obligatory diversity training; migrant-specific family planning;[8] establishing multi-religious spaces in hospitals; and employment of migrant staff. Suggestions by interviewees from Leipzig included: culturally sensitive geriatric care; engagement of community cultural translators based in the municipality in bigger cities; expansion of curricula addressing health care and diversity for medical students (medical anthropology); cultural mediators in health offices; sensitization of migrant school children; emphasizing programs for female cultural mediators and translators (especially for maternity care); translators and cultural mediators whose costs are legally covered by the city or health insurance; emergency meetings; sensitization of people in high, powerful positions; focusing on prevention programs; legislating translation services; and protecting migrants in psychiatric care from deportation.

While the hospital staff interviewed in Leipzig are partly in favor of migrant-specific services, these services hardly exist. The only migrant-specific services available are multilingual flyers in three languages and the ambulant psychiatric service for ethnic Germans organized by one of the state-owned hospitals (*Städtisches Klinikum St. Georg*). Practitioners explain the low level of sensitivity toward increasing services geared for migrants' specific needs as related to a low migrant density in Leipzig, as well as a lack of information and time. A professional working on prenatal and maternity care in Leipzig noted that:

> there is no contact point. The best would be if we would have contact information [through translators and cultural mediators] because they are equipped with specific tools to provide specific help. That would be very helpful for doctors

7 Interviewees in Leipzig remained rather vague about the implementation of migrant-friendly services. While arguing that medical care is being adjusted to specific culturally-conditioned gender sensitivities and that religion "is being considered," they never specified about the different methods. There is one hospital in Leipzig with a multi-religious prayer room. Overall, it can be concluded that migrant-specific services hardly exist in Leipzig hospitals and if at all are reflected in the context of economizing strategies.

8 This was mentioned in light of very high abortion rates among migrant women.

> who could then focus on their medical help. (Department Head, Prenatal and Birth Medicine, hospital, Leipzig, 2007)

While the BoH in Bremen has long established two permanent doctors in asylum homes, the BoH in Leipzig has recently begun to consider offering such services, as argued by a BoH employee:

> I argued recently in the Social Security Office to establish a medical care institution for asylum seekers. If they would need a specialized practitioner they would be connected. In a similar manner we could also provide health care for homeless people. Both are difficult clients and have lots in common. (Health Office, Leipzig, 2007)

In the German case studies, there were two central narrative strategies in which arguments about the ICO of the health care system were couched. The first relates to expanding the existing quality management system for patient interviews by including migrant-specific issues. Clinic directors were explicit about their commitment to improving the quality of care with migrant-specific services (Medical Board Hospital, Leipzig 2006). The second relates to the fact that migrant-specific strategies are not framed in a context of patients' rights, the quality of care or a medical or moral ethos; instead they are framed as a strategy for institutions to overcome financial challenges. As suggested by a health policy expert interested in attracting migrant patients to their service: "Care providers and [departments] that compete with each other could procure an advantage if they use migration as a marketing tool" (health policy expert, Leipzig, 2006). This narrative highlights and justifies improved access and services for migrants with a market-oriented rationale, emphasizing the economic imperatives under which health care systems increasingly have to operate.

The Political and Regulatory Framework in Canada

There are various legal provisions in Canada at the federal level, and in both British Columbia (BC) and Québec at the provincial level, which set the legal framework for intercultural opening (ICO) in the governing of different policy fields. The Canadian (Government of Canada 1982) and Québec (Quebec 1975) Charters of Human Rights and Freedoms and the BC Human Rights Code (British Columbia 1996b) explicitly protect against racial discrimination in employment and service access. The Multiculturalism Act of Canada (Government of Canada 1988) and the BC Multiculturalism Act (British Columbia 1996a) both guarantee the commitment to equality through promoting inclusion in social life. The BC Multiculturalism Act states that it is the government's role to "foster the ability of each British Columbian, regardless of race, cultural heritage, religion, ethnicity, ancestry or place of origin, to share in the economic, social, cultural and political life of British Columbia" (British Columbia 1996a). The Multiculturalism Act of Canada contains even stronger language about the role of ethnically diverse communities, explicitly stating that it is federal policy to "promote the full and equitable participation of individuals and communities of all origins in the continuing evolution and shaping of all aspects of Canadian society and assist them in the elimination of any barrier to that participation" (Government of Canada 1988). The BC Human Rights Code of 1996 is also a tool that can be used to protect the rights of ethnic minority communities. Specifically with reference to service provision, the BC Human Rights Code states that:

> [n]o person, without a bona fide and reasonable justification, shall a) deny to a person or class of persons any accommodation, service or facility customarily available to the public, or b) discriminate against a person or class of persons with respect to any accommodation, service or facility customarily available to the public, because of the race, colour, ancestry, place of origin, religion, marital status, family status, physical or mental disability, sex or sexual orientation of that person or class of persons. (British Columbia 1996b)

Similarly, the Québec Charter of Human Rights and Freedoms supports the rights of ethnic minority people. The Québec Charter states that:

> [e]very person has a right to full and equal recognition and exercise of his human rights and freedoms, without distinction, exclusion or preference based on race, colour, sex, pregnancy, sexual orientation, civil status, age except as provided by law, religion, political convictions, language, ethnic or national origin, social condition, a handicap or the use of any means to palliate a handicap. Discrimination exists where such a distinction, exclusion or preference has the effect of nullifying or impairing such right. (Québec 1975)

Health care in Canada is federally legislated based on principles of universality, accessibility, portability, comprehensiveness and public administration; however, its delivery is under the jurisdiction of the provincial governments. In Québec (hence in Montreal), the mandate of the Ministry of Health and Social Services is legislated in the Act Respecting Health and Social Services. This Act explicitly states a number of assurances for ethnocultural communities. The law states that "[t]he health services and social services plan established by this Act aims to maintain and improve the physical, mental and social capacity of persons to act in their community and to carry out the roles they intend to assume in a manner which is acceptable to themselves and to the groups to which they belong," and continues to note that this plan will cover "the various strata of the population and in the various regions" while "attaining comparable standards of health and welfare." Moreover, the law also prioritizes the "participation of individuals and groups of individuals in the selection of orientations and in the setting up, improvement, development and management of services." The "services are accessible on a continuous basis to respond to the physical, mental and social needs of individuals, families and groups." All of these parameters will also take into consideration "the distinctive geographical, linguistic, sociocultural, ethnocultural and socioeconomic characteristics of each region" with the aim of facilitating access "to the extent allowed by the resources" (Québec 2010: Section 1 and 2).

In addition to the guarantees outlined above, Bill 83 was brought into law in the Act Respecting Health and Social Services in 2005 and led to the establishment of the Committee for the Dispensation of Health and Social Services to Persons of Ethnocultural Communities (Québec 2010: Section 433.1). This committee provides advice and recommendations on policy, and also works to identify priority issues for Québec's many ethnocultural communities.

In a 2006 national report on the health status of the population, the Government of Québec explicitly states that poverty and social exclusion have a significant impact on health and needs to be addressed (Québec 2006a). A 2006 report in Québec notes that health and social services are founded upon principles of social justice and equity (Québec 2006b). A Québec public health report clearly states that "social solidarity allows us to take into account the specific needs of groups or individuals who have more problems or risk factors," identifies ethnic minorities as communities that are vulnerable and calls for a balance between universal measures and selective measures targeting vulnerable groups (Québec 2003: 20–21).

The *Montreal Agence* (regional health authority) is responsible for delivering health services on the Island of Montreal, a population of approximately 1.9 million people, which is about 25 percent of the population of Québec. The population in this area is ethnically diverse, with a large proportion speaking languages other than French or English. The *Montreal Agence* also states that the accessibility of health services for ethnocultural communities is an integral part of their work, which aims to break down communication barriers and support intercultural training of managers and workers (Santé Montreal 2004).

In BC, the Provincial Health Services Authority offers a variety of interpretation, translation and training services to help health organizations across BC provide better services to ethnically and linguistically diverse populations. Regional Health Authorities (RHAs) are responsible for the delivery of care within regional boundaries, from hospitals to community-based health services to public health and health promotion activities. The provincial government signs accountability contracts with the RHAs regarding the services that they are to provide and the financial resources for those services. The service contracts between the Ministry of Health and the Vancouver Coastal Health Authority states that: "The health authority will … provide services that meet the priority health needs of the population of the health authority within its available budget" (British Columbia 2005: 2). Vancouver Coastal Health Authority (VCH) is responsible for the city of Vancouver and coastal communities across a relatively small geographic area with a high population density. VCH serves just over one million people, which is 25 percent of the population of BC and one of the most ethnically diverse regions in Canada.

VCH has a variety of multicultural service programs, including outreach, health promotion, maternity care and provision of translation services on site at the Vancouver General Hospital. Many patient information materials are available in multiple languages. The Bridge Clinic was established in 1994 and provides services to any newly-arrived refugee or refugee claimant. As the Bridge Clinic brochure notes, "the name 'Bridge' conveys the clinic's mandate to provide a bridge or temporary transition to medical services in the Vancouver area" (Vancouver Coastal Health n.d.: 2). In addition, VCH has a department dedicated to community engagement. Its aim is to promote "a formalized approach for gathering feedback from the public," which is constituted of "clients, patients, residents and other community stakeholders," in order "to improve decisions and ensure that the system is responsive to their concerns" (Vancouver Coastal Health 2005: 1).

Civil Society Actors Interacting with Health Care System in Canada

In Montreal, community groups focused a lot of their work on raising awareness within health services institutions "to promote the understanding of diversity as being a primary concern, and that the health care institutions have to adapt to that" (representative, Migrant Association, Montreal, 2006). This includes preparing statements to governments about the issues communities face, particularly where there are service gaps, such as in mental health. In addition, community groups provide information sessions for their members on the services available and how to access them through weekly open houses and ongoing presentations involving health service providers. Many community groups will accompany clients if they need support when accessing health services. For example, a community women's organization together with local health and social service centers known as CLSCs (*centres de santé et de services sociaux*), initiated a project aimed at addressing the mental health of immigrant women to help address the isolation and lack of participation in civil life that is common for many immigrant women.

ACCÉSSS (*Alliance des communautés culturelles pour l'égalité dans la santé et les services sociaux*), an umbrella association that brings together a variety of community organizations, has become more involved with training and services. For example, ACCÉSSS works with various groups of women from immigrant communities around cancer prevention. In addition, they do work with nutrition, diet and sensitizing women about other health issues, such as weight, baby weight, food security, nutrition and sexuality. They also focus on improving understanding of the mental health issues that immigrants and refugees face, particularly those from war-torn areas (ACCÉSSS 2006, 2007).

In Vancouver, we also see information partnerships between community associations and health service providers. For example the health authority will send staff to participate in English as a Second Language (ESL) courses so that they can provide information to newcomers about the services available. One of the most significant ongoing partnerships is the Multicultural Health Fair, which is hosted by the Affiliation of Multicultural Societies and Service Agencies (AMSSA) in collaboration with the health authorities, community health centers, other health service providers and community associations. This fair takes place every year, and all groups participating need to offer multilingual interactive activities (AMSSA 2004).

There is a considerable amount of collaboration between the health care system and community associations in providing multicultural health promotion programs. For example, there are diabetes education programs offered in Cantonese, Mandarin and Farsi, and a multicultural healthy eating campaign aimed at seniors. Other programs address food security issues through community kitchens and nutritional counseling for ethnic communities. An immigrant settlement worker explained that they offer:

> a number of programs for immigrant youth—children and youth—that involve training modules in … mental health … We have an 80-hour leadership facilitation-training program for immigrant youth which has a big section on mental health, where we have guest speakers coming in. So [we are] increasing the capacity of youth to deal with not only their own mental health concerns or issues, but also to be better support for incoming youth in their schools or neighbourhoods. (Immigrant settlement worker, Vancouver, 2006)

In the Canadian case, for both Vancouver and Montreal community organizations and liaison workers play a critical role in improving access to health care services. Their main strategy is to act as guides for navigating through the health care system.

The role of migrant associations in Montreal is critical in terms of facilitating access to information about different services available to immigrants. One of the members of the associations interviewed states that their role as guides surfaces when they inform those who recently arrived in Montreal not only about health services, but also about "social services, and also education, employability, even consumption" (representative, Migrant Association, Montreal, 2006). This facilitates the recent immigrants' knowledge about how to use the system for their different social and economic needs.

Migrant associations receive requests from patients from ethnocultural communities concerning how they may navigate the system:

> Our clients tell us that they don't know how to do something, and we send a volunteer … Very often, the person asks for us to go with them. Either they do not speak sufficiently, or they say that they aren't really familiar with [how the service works] and [ask]: 'can we come [with them]?' (Representative, Migrant Association, Montreal, 2006)

Alternatively, staff in the health care system also count on the support of migrant associations in Montreal regarding the challenges they encounter while delivering services to patients of different ethnic backgrounds: "Many times, like CLSC-Metro, CLSC-Côte-des-Neiges, they call [us] to give … information with reference [to] the culture—how to deal with patients when they are from this community, how to approach them, how to get information" (representative, Migrant Association, Montreal, 2006).

Both the health care providers and the patients use the migrant associations as facilitators for overcoming diversity-related challenges. At the same time, different actors in the health care system recognize the value of collaboration among the ethnocultural groups and the health care system. An example of such partnerships on mental health initiatives would be between women's organizations and the CLSCs in Parc-Extension and Côte-des-Neiges, which are both located in ethnically diverse neighborhoods. Through this partnership, women in the diverse community work with health centers to promote solutions to women's health matters. Reflecting on the sustainability of such initiatives for solving problems in the system, one staff member suggested that further progress may be achieved "if everybody gets involved, comes to know … what is available here and what these people are going through" (representative, Migrant Association, Montreal, 2006). In other words, those who work on such initiatives value the benefits of cooperation among the stakeholders for overcoming challenges of access. Therefore, the extent to which health centers are equipped with knowledge about diverse groups (in this case, the social context of women's lives in ethnically diverse communities) and their possible needs in the system shapes the extent to which community health access may improve. Such collaboration promotes access to the health care system as a whole by enhancing knowledge of one part of the system through collaboration.

Migrant-Specific Services in Montreal and Vancouver

In Montreal, the organization of health and social services as part of the same institution facilitates access to a number of services by different immigrant communities. As they are informed by this network, they are highly likely to be able to access and use various different services even after their first arrival. As one staff member highlights, such linking between service providers and immigrants is praised by migrant associations: "Québec does a good job in terms of informing the new arrivals about the health care structure. If you have a problem … you have a variety of channels" (representative, Migrant Association, Montreal, 2006).

In contrast to the approach observed in Montreal, in Vancouver the approach to facilitating access to the health care system for ethnically diverse communities is more formalized through the use of liaison workers. For example, health settlement workers provide general information on the health care system and suggest specific services for migrants based on his/her ethnic background (including linking patients with a doctor that can speak their language). Since in principle the

Bridge Clinic would be the first encounter newcomers have with the health care system, the clinic would also pass along medical histories to newcomers' doctors for appropriate follow-up for patients with health concerns. The services of the Bridge Clinic are predominantly for the three month period in which immigrants wait to be eligible for the medical services program or to those who are waiting for a decision on their refugee claims.

In addition to the health settlement workers, VCH funded a pilot program to provide liaison workers who can accompany the patient throughout the health care system. These liaison workers:

> do more than just interpreting. These are people who are bilingual and largely bi-cultural. They largely come from medical backgrounds in their home countries and they will accompany a patient through the health care system. So [while] an interpreter just comes in for that one hour appointment with the doctor, the health broker will follow the patient through various health care settings and help them not [just] understand what the doctor is physically saying, but the meaning of what is being said as well—so they'll help with advice, advocacy, some support. And they'll also help the doctors, so it'll become really a three-way conversation. Now, they're not there to give medical advice, but they're there to support the patients, so the patient is actually empowered to make their own decisions. (Liaison worker, Vancouver, 2006)

The liaison project started in the 1990s as a partnership between various health care service organizations. Its initial goal was to provide peri-natal support services, partly to assist in the hospital's aim to reduce the length of stay after giving birth. These facilitators accompany patients through the health care system and the various services they use in the system. The overall aim was for this program to increase the appropriate use of health care services and ensure that patients get appropriate care:

> These clients have so many different problems—they come with more complications: they will be misdiagnosed, have delayed diagnosis, unnecessary hospitalization, unnecessary, inappropriate referral to specialists or … diagnostic tests. [The health liaison worker] will reduce the pressure and the burden financially on the health care system. The health care provider will have more time … because the communication will be facilitated … and their patients have better health outcomes and support, and increased access to services. (Liaison worker, Vancouver, 2006)

The liaison workers project also transformed from its initial focus on the facilitation of appropriate service use to a partnership with immigrant settlement services organizations. Some of their work includes training migrant associations about the types of health services available, how to access them and how to identify mental health issues that their community members may be experiencing. In addition, facilitators are provided with training about the various kinds of services available in addition to health services, such as processes for obtaining a health care card and information about housing, day-care, schooling, counseling and other services which largely affect health. As one of the coordinators of the health liaison workers project explained:

> For example, if your client has a problem with housing, … if there is a problem with day-care, [the] medical service plan, health insurance, or schooling, counseling—all those things—we try to cover a lot of different things, like non-medical determinants of health and resources available … We had a session for them about Canadian health care, the people in the health care system, the [Canada] Health Act and the rights of the patients … We had the training about palliative care and hospice because it was a new term and new idea for them. (Liaison worker, Vancouver, 2006)

In both Montreal and Vancouver, several clinics and programs provide services specifically for immigrants and refugees to improve access to health care services for diverse communities. In Montreal, the Montreal Children's Hospital (MCH) and various community health services are particularly geared toward multicultural care. Additionally, maternity care services aim to address the needs of diverse communities more effectively when compared to other areas of health. The respondents interviewed in our study noted that in both Montreal and Vancouver, pediatrics and maternity care are the two areas which advance multicultural health care provision. The MCH was identified by many respondents as one of the most responsive institutions for addressing the needs of the multicultural community in Montreal. The MCH has offered a multicultural program for over 20 years and has established a reputation which attracts most of the diverse communities to this hospital to receive care. The staff is also trained in cross-cultural care, and provides comprehensive services including education and training, as well as a multicultural library. A hospital based service provider noted that the hospital based services can provide more comprehensive care for newcomers:

> People who are new to the country are coming in and maybe don't have very clear medical histories—that they're not documented. In the multicultural clinic, they take very detailed medical histories and get to know the families, and provide services where other CLSCs cannot or don't know how to really get into it because it's too overwhelming for them. That's what they say. Whereas here every effort is made to ensure that the person's health is checked, the child's health is checked and that families have what they need within the context of a hospital service (Diversity program staff, hospital, Montreal 2006).

There are also a few community health centers (CLSCs—now grouped into the CSSS) that stand out as particularly welcoming of diversity, due to the nature of the population within their service areas. In one area, approximately 80 languages are spoken and the health center has been addressing diversity and health care access issues for over a decade, and they have a number of documents that address issues of immigrant health to help professionals know about the challenges linked to immigration. These efforts and documents adopt a comprehensive approach to health whereby they relate matters of immigration to issues such as poverty, and economic and social exclusion. The CSSS also launched a research program that addresses immigration and ethnicity towards a practice of inclusive citizenship, and health practices to adapt to diversity.

In prenatal care, there have been multiple initiatives aimed at meeting the needs of women from ethnocultural communities. These efforts have taken place within community and health authority partnerships, such as multi-lingual pre-natal services to address the need among immigrant women. Another CLSC has a birthing house that provides services to their diverse community. Such practices originate mostly from the needs of the diverse population and are intensified by the concentrated presence of the community in the area. As noted by a staff member of the birthing house: "You have to adjust. You can't really say: 'Okay, we do our copy of the Québec perception of giving birth.' So you have to adapt … It's less difficult for us, because [cultural adaptation is part of] our philosophy" (midwife, community clinic, Montreal, 2006). Similarly, a maternal health clinic situated near Chinatown receives requests for high-risk pregnancy clinics in Mandarin and Cantonese. Such demands also increase in relation to the follow-ups required for high-risk pregnant women and their babies.

The Bridge Clinic in Vancouver constitutes an exemplar in facilitating access to health services for new immigrants and refugees. The clinic was established in 1994 with the aim of providing access to primary and preventative health care services for immigrants and refugees. This clinic serves new immigrants and refugees for their first year in Vancouver, although some patients stay longer. The clinic aims to bridge people into other health care services, help them acquire their health care cards and locate a family doctor. The practitioners speak a variety of languages and include physicians, nurses, interpreters, settlement workers, nutritionists, a physiotherapist, a speech language pathologist, a psychologist and a psychiatrist. These specialty services include prenatal care, the Newcomer's Pediatric Health Clinic, chronic disease management, immigration medical examinations, mental health services, nutritional counseling, physiotherapy, respiratory therapy and speech language pathology.

The rationale behind establishing the Bridge Clinic was to help new immigrants and refugees adapt to the health care system with more ease. The health authority has re-structured some of the operations of the Bridge Clinic to make it more cost effective, making such adjustments as moving health assessment exams to another agency and advocating for patients to be moved through more quickly to connect with other services.

Another good example of helping diverse communities with peri-natal care similar to Montreal is through a community birthing project. This project involves a multidisciplinary team of physicians, midwives, nurses and doulas, with staff representing a diversity of ethnic groups. While establishing the program, they have aimed to overcome the challenge posed by the cost of translators by training doulas with multilingual skills in order to provide care in the mother tongue of many of their clients:

> One of the things that we really wanted to do was to provide translation, language services but, as you probably know, it's prohibitively expensive to get translators. So we trained our own doulas ... Right now we have 14 different language groups, so all of our doulas are bilingual ... So then we match them—say if their language is Punjabi, then we match them with a Punjabi-speaking woman, so then they also can translate for us, of course not as an official translator, but certainly as a communicator for the woman. Even if the woman speaks English, sometimes it's more comfortable for her in labour to communicate in Punjabi, so we can get the information from the doula. (Midwife, community clinic, Vancouver, 2006)

The doulas attend the birth so that the mother will have someone there for her with whom she can communicate. In addition, similar to emphasizing the need to focus also on social determinants of health in Montreal, Vancouver runs a program called Healthiest Babies Possible (HBP), which targets low income women and offers services in a variety of languages. HBP was started in the early 1980s, although funding has declined for these programs in recent years. Therefore, in both Vancouver and Montreal, there are institutional initiatives that introduce and partially support existing and new structures to advance health service delivery for diverse communities.

Unlike Québec, where interpreters are available for the entire health and social services network, in Vancouver interpretation services offered by the health authority have been limited to some hospital services and the Bridge Clinic. This program meets over 5000 annual requests for interpretation and provides staff training on working with interpreters. Therefore the main virtue of this program is that it is at no cost to the specific departments or patients. In Vancouver there is also a specialized interpreter training program provided through the Vancouver Community College. The interpretation services in the hospital are available within 24 hours, although it is often a shorter waiting period for the dominant language groups (Punjabi and Chinese languages). The Provincial Health Services Authority also operates an interpreter services program that offers these services in its areas of jurisdiction, such as the BC Women's Hospital and the Children's Hospital. The services are available for over 100 languages, primarily through telephone interpretation, so as one interviewee noted: "in theory, you should never be without, if you need it" (Diversity program manager, hospital, Vancouver, 2006).

There is published material on health care services in multiple languages available in Vancouver. The BC Health Guide is published in Chinese, Punjabi and Farsi, and there are over 300 patient education materials translated. The translation for documentation comes from program budgets, limiting the ability to update materials or translate into other languages, as the money for this would need to be taken out of service delivery costs. The Nurseline, a telephone health service, has over 130 languages available, as does the BC Dial-a-Dietician telephone service. Vancouver General Hospital also has signage in Chinese and Punjabi. In Vancouver there are also language designated public health nurse positions that match language groups with the characteristic of the local population, with designated positions for Chinese, Punjabi and Spanish speaking nurses.

The respondents of our study pointed to intercultural training of health care personnel as a key way of ensuring that the health care system would facilitate the construction of a welcoming environment for culturally diverse populations. In both Vancouver and Montreal, workshops on intercultural training are available for staff in the health care system, although there are often limited resources to be able to dedicate staff time to these training programs.

The Ministry of Health and Social Services (MSSS) of Québec provides support for the adaptation of institutions to deliver services to the culturally diverse populations by intercultural training for the network of practitioners, offering approximately 65 intercultural training courses over 2003–06. These courses have differing content based on the needs identified across the themes of access, engagement as well as social determinants of health. Since 1997 the MSSS has provided consultants who carry out the training to institution managers, who are then responsible for training their staff and adapting services according to the needs of their diverse clientele. The health service delivery institutions are currently responsible to initiate intercultural training, either on their own or via requests to the MSSS.

The hospital multicultural programs constitute a major resource for intercultural training with a library and regular intercultural training sessions. A program manager describes their practices as follows:

> We give workshops and presentations on working across cultures, on anti-racism. We design sessions specifically to meet the needs of the teams that we're speaking to—whether it's nurses or genetic counselors or occupational therapists or doctors. Next week I have to go and give a presentation in emergency. So [I will focus on] some of the kinds of issues that come up in emergency. (Diversity program manager, hospital, Montreal, 2006)

In the health care system in Montreal, there is commitment to training and awareness raising on needs of culturally diverse communities in health care. Many institutions provide intercultural training manuals to their staff which cover issues such as health and diverse religions, death, mourning and grieving and diverse societies. However this commitment is not always matched by allocation of resources. In such circumstances the institutions relay on volunteer students to produce intercultural material. Intercultural/multicultural health committees constitute another strategy for the enhancement of cultural understanding among staff, where health professionals and intern students discuss intercultural matters and academic material to enhance their capacity to work with culturally diverse communities. Such committees also provide a good opportunity to compare and engage with academic research by drawing from daily practice. A significantly different approach to learning about working with cultural groups in the health care system is practiced in a hospital in Montreal through multidisciplinary intervention groups. This unique practice is composed of pediatricians, anthropologists, and psychiatrists that according to one health care professional assists providers to:

> understand why the situation evolved in a negative way … But it's never by giving an answer. It's by giving clues and they make their path … When an exchange is made, like for example in a service unit where I made observations … I was told after a year that there were changes. That is, they think about things about which they are not used to thinking, and it has a snow-ball effect, which provokes, what we call the reflective effect of research. And it works. (Diversity program manager, hospital, Montreal, 2006)

Despite all these strategies aiming to raise awareness and generate know-how for accommodating different needs in the health care system emanating from diversity, discrepancies may be observed in the system as a whole. For example, in Montreal, the Francophone institutions display a higher demand for training and for interpreters than the Anglophone ones. One explanation for this could be the nature of the immigration policy of Québec which promotes the arrival of French speaking communities and also supports learning French in integration classes after arrival. Therefore most of the new comers to Québec (hence Montreal) tend to utilize health services available in French or through Francophone institutions. The staff's commitment to training also wavers, some are more eager to participate than others. The intercultural training is more widely available in Montreal advancing in the 2000s, and also spreading out to also other regions in Québec to which immigrants began to move.

Intercultural training has also been increasingly incorporated to the formal curricula for medical students. For example, UQAM has a compulsory course for the senior year on approaches to culturally diverse clientele in the health care system; the University of Montreal also started a new intercultural training program. The training provided on communication skills has also been adapted to account for the needs of the diverse groups.

In Vancouver, the diversity programs provide intercultural training through staff orientation sessions. They also provide handbooks on working across cultures. One of the key themes for the cross-cultural education in the diversity services program in Vancouver is to provide tools to assist the health care providers to understand the need to go beyond stereotypes in their dealings with patients from another culture:

> Around the cross-cultural care piece, a lot of times what people want is … cultural profiles. The trouble with the cultural profiles is that they have a very

> limited [value] … So what I try to do is … talk about the intersections of ethnicity, migration history and some of the social issues like education, class, marriage status, all that kind of stuff … And then, because people are so keen on cultural profiles … we do an exercise with cultural profiles, and help them see what is useful in a cultural profile and what's not useful, because there are some that are actually good … So we do an exercise with them on that … I give them a cultural profile, give them a case study, and … say how is this person like their culture, and how are they different? (Diversity program manager, hospital, Vancouver, 2006)

Immigrant service organizations also perform a significant role in advancing strategies for influencing change in the health care system in Vancouver. For example, immigrant settlement services make presentations to health authorities which serve the purpose of:

> providing background contextual information for new communities to give people a heads up on what they're dealing with—what they're going to see. And it helps then for their own internal program planning and in-service training. (Immigrant settlement worker, Vancouver, 2006)

Comparing the role of health practitioners and liaison workers in Montreal and Vancouver reveals many similarities. The first is the pattern of evolving partnerships among the different associations and health care providers functioning within the system. All of the health care staff and representatives of associations emphasize the value of such partnerships for improving access to services with a global approach. The endorsement of appropriate access to health services depends not only on overcoming the challenges around specific access issues (such as overcoming language barriers or lack of knowledge about the system), but also on addressing challenges around social determinants of health. Second, there is also a pattern whereby migrant associations support improved access by linking those in need of services with health care providers. The third pattern is the will and commitment in the system to address these challenges through collaboration among health care providers and those working in support services to newcomers, as well as among ethnocultural communities themselves. The main difference is that while the Montreal case relies on more informal partnerships formed and sustained by pioneers in the system, the Vancouver case introduces more formal models for partnerships in the field of health care. However, neither case provides a panacea for the sustainability of these efforts.

The Political and Regulatory Framework in Italy

In order to understand the strategies for change that Italian civil society actors have pursued, one has to identify the distinctive aspects of the Italian policy and political environment that affect them. In particular, a complex interaction is taking place between ideology, a regulatory system of universalist entitlements, territorial fragmentation, a highly differentiated availability of resources and an unequal distribution of social capital in different areas of the country. Thus, after a review of the main traits of the institutional and legal systems, we will discuss the differentiated strategies of organized civil society in the two case studies of Trento and Naples.

Italy's health care system is a regionally-based national health system that provides universal coverage. The Italian Constitution recognizes the right to the protection of health for every individual as a fundamental right and as an interest of the community, guaranteeing free care to people in need. Every person has the right to assistance from the national health system, or "*Servizio Sanitario Nazionale*" (NHS). Everyone can, in addition, add a private health care plan to cover expenses not covered by the NHS. Everyone is entitled to choose a general practitioner from a public list that guarantees basic care free of charge. Users always need a general practitioner consultation prior to obtaining prescriptions and referrals to specialists. To receive treatments in hospitals (e.g., specialist visits, exams), one must pay a ticket at subsidized prices. One can also opt for private practitioners or clinics whose prices are higher but do not have long waiting lists.

Institutions and actors in the NHS and its decision-making political referents are organized in three levels of government: The national level includes Parliament, which approves health legislation and defines available resources annually; the Ministry of Health, which operates in conjunction with various technical and consultative commissions and establishes the three year National Health Plan (*Piano Sanitario Nazionale*, PSN); and the government, which approves the National Health Plan. The second level is the regional level. This includes the Government-Regions Conference (Conferenza Stato-Regioni), which establishes the regional allocation of financial resources, and the regions, which approve the regional health legislation that establishes the three year Regional Health Plan (*Piano Sanitario Regionale*, PSR). The regional level legislates the local allocation of financial resources and elects the directors of the Local Health Units. Due to a recent constitutional reform, regions now have legislative power with regard to health issues, while the state sets fundamental principles and guarantees homogenous standards and/ or levels of performance and services. The third level is the local level. This includes Local Health Units, which organize the various services that supply medical care at the local level: general practitioners, public hospitals and health care providers covered by the public health insurance.

In recent years, the NHS adopted a policy of territorial fragmentation of services with the aim of becoming more responsive to the health needs of the population. Specifically, Act 229/99 reformed the Healthcare Service and Act 328/2000 reformed the welfare system by introducing the concept of integration of health and social services. These acts also established a new model of policy based on the principle of subsidiarity, which redesigns the system with the aim of providing integrated competences and responsibilities at the level closest to local administrative units (i.e., health districts, councils, provinces). By identifying the local area as a fundamental unit of service delivery and the context in which local decisions are made, the direct intervention of citizens is promoted with the intention of stimulating participation and transparency for public choices (Sasci 2003). However, at the same time, the growing political autonomy of all Italian regions increases territorial differentiation among regional health systems. In theory, every region could modify the universalist principles of the NHS. Therefore, there is a dynamic tension between the national government seeking to keep a role of coordination and control and the regions asserting their administrative autonomy.

By 2000, a set of new legislative norms (Legislative Degree 56/2000 and the Pact of internal stability—*Patto di stabilità interna*) increasingly decentralized the collection of revenues. On the one hand, this involved enhanced financial autonomy for the regions. On the other, it forced the regions to observe norms of financial probity mandated at the European level. The general goal of decreasing Italy's public deficit now involves a direct role for the regions, which are obliged to contain health expenditures. Although an agreement that obliges the government to increase regional resources has been signed between the state and the regions, there is tension between the two levels of government concerning responsibilities for past debts and with regard to who can authorize increases of current expenditures. Some regions (e.g., Lazio, Campania and Sicily) have a huge deficit and this fact implies a higher risk of territorial differentiation among regional health systems. This general normative framework has important implications for immigrants' access to the health system, as the general wealth, fiscal probity and administrative efficiency of different regions have a growing impact on all policy sectors, including the health sector. There are, however, historical legacies with regard to how migrants are conceptualized that also come to play a relevant role.

Before the collapse of the first republic in the early 1990s, Italian political culture was split between two universalisms (Communist and Catholic) and refused to make political use of internal ethnic rivalries. In that context, migrants and their needs were supported by existing political discourse. In fact, to simplify a multifaceted issue, one could have seen migrants as ideally incorporated by the Left in the general category of the international proletariat and by the Church as part of its social mission of supporting the poor. With the collapse of the party system following a set of corruption scandals, the situation changed. Capitalizing upon and fuelling ethnic tensions, the ethno-nationalist 'Northern League' movement began to acquire electoral support by thematizing and politicizing a Northern Italian territorial identity that was previously merely cultural. As internal migration abated, the language of ethnic discrimination changed (Ruzza and Schmidtke 1996). Parties of the Right profited from the fears engendered by migration. A content analysis of party documents reveals an increasingly negative focus on migration over the last decade (Fella and Ruzza 2006). It is in this context that migration began to be conceptualized as a security issue. In 1998, even the center-left government approved a framework law to regulate migration policy: the Turco-Napolitano law, which instituted special temporary holding camps (CPTs—centri di permanenzatemporanea) to detain illegal immigrants. After the 2001 election, the center-right replaced the center-left government and took a more exclusionary stand on migration-related issues. As mentioned in previous chapters, this stance was characterized by a new law on immigration—the Bossi-Fini law—which attempted to clamp down on clandestine immigration and tied legal immigration to the possession of employment contracts. However, notwithstanding the negative framing of the migration issue by some political forces, migrants are now a well-established and economically necessary presence in Italy. The specificity of migrants as a sub-sector of the population is decreasing as they become a better integrated component of the Italian population. Their numbers are now considerable for a country that, until recently, has had a low presence of migrants. The number of foreign citizens present in 2009 was over four million, which is equal to 7.2 percent of the Italian population. Two million are regular workers and 862,000 are minors who were born from foreign parents. In this context, illegal arrivals now amount to only 1 percent of the foreign population, pointing to the fact that the issue of clandestine migration is often excessively accentuated in the media and by political actors (Caritas Italiana—Fondazione Migrantes 2010).

Thus, to summarize, the distinctive features of the Italian regulatory environment are those of a system which acts on the basis of universalist principles, but in a context of widely different resources across the regions and widely different political cultures. In this context, the universalist principles of the law are not homogenously implemented in different locations. Finally, in order to understand the issue of state attitudes toward intercultural representation, it should be pointed out that the Italian state has historically been fashioned according to the principles of a strong state that is closed to non-state actors of the Napoleonic type. It is not then a state that historically conceives its role as one of mediating among different types of territorial representations of interests easily. Rather, Italy is a state closed to external interests, which are conceived as particularistic intrusions. This closure has been modified in recent years by two emerging ideologies. As previously mentioned, on the one hand, the principles of *New Public Management* have required an opening of state structures to societal actors in order to improve information exchanges and therefore effectiveness. On the other hand, a focus on participation as part of a more deliberative vision of the role of democratic institutions is also gaining momentum.

However, both the earlier state closure to external influences and the successive attempts at reform in the direction of more openness have been filtered by a *de facto* practice of receptivity to corporatist interests, which are evaluated in terms of their perceived social power and to an extent in terms of their perceived social representativeness. Thus, public bureaucracies tend to take the role of adjudicators among conflicting interests, rather than implementers of a vision—any vision—of the good society, which would require, for instance, that weak groups carrying marginalized but legitimate social interests are appropriately supported. Therefore, the fact that migrants' associations are in principle in need of support (given the social relevance or the poverty of these constituencies) is not conceptualized as an appropriate consideration. This point is, for instance, reflected in an interview with a local councilor:

> With associations it is necessary to be very attentive. I believe that it is also necessary to be very open. I mean that sometimes migrants speaking on behalf of their association claim to speak on behalf of their entire community. This is often not the case. However, even if a person does not necessarily represent the community, he might represent a section of the community. So, in such a situation becoming uncritically supportive of the opinions represented by a person and not worrying about the others would be wrong, as it would create dissatisfaction in the rest of the community. I think that our job is to become aware of the entire reality through contacts with associations and their representatives. So this is necessary in order to act appropriately. First we have to focus on knowing what is happening. Our primary task is one of knowing. We are a complex system that interacts with a myriad of associations. All carriers of interests need to be listened to. But then of course we take the decisions. So we relate to these associations as we relate to the associations of Italians, such as the diabetic association, or the association of hospital assistants. We focus on creating mechanisms of consultation which are comprehensive and collective. (City councilor, Trento, 2006)

In this interview, one senses that there is goodwill and a desire to learn to produce good policies. One also sees a preoccupation with issues of accountability and representativeness. However, there is no indication that the difficulties of migrants, as a vulnerable social constituency, are taken in full consideration. They are seen as just another interest group within a framework in which inequalities in social power and the constitutionalized need to promote integration of all citizens are not paramount.

Migrant Specific Services in Italy

In Italy various strategies have been pursued to improve the health situation of migrants. As has been previously pointed out there is a substantial difference of planning capacity, organizational effectiveness and network effectiveness between Trento and Naples. Consequently, there are more instances of new and promising approaches in Trento. We will review some of the key examples of innovation. Possibly the most relevant factor in promoting institutional openness in Trento has been the dedicated support by areas of civil society which are internal to the medical profession. Success in improving health services to migrants has drawn upon the skilled use of the social prestige and general societal legitimacy that doctors enjoy in a traditional and corporatist society such as Italy. In this context, the work of GRIS—a civil society organization previously discussed and based on the volunteering activities of doctors in Trento—has been particularly influential because of their social status, as several interviewees have pointed out. Doctors have also been successfully involved in promoting distinctive service delivery initiatives, such as their effort to liaise with medical personnel in the countries of origin. This is particularly important when an area is facing temporary migration patterns in which migrants spend part of the year in the host country and part in the native country. This is for instance often the case of careers for older people in Trento ('*badanti*') who tend to be early middle aged women who come from Eastern Europe for several months each year but also return home fairly frequently for family and health care reasons. Here the necessity to connect services received in the home country and services in Italy is essential and members of GRIS have been particularly effective. Thus committed doctors are important both in their advocacy efforts and in their service delivery activities.

One area that has been identified as in need of attention is a better connection between the policy shaping activities that civil society can offer and public institutions. There is a need to effectively channel the expertise that civil society has acquired to support organizational structuring and service implementation. In this context, Trento has been at the forefront of connecting service delivery and policy shaping through a planned consultation of migrants and their organizations. Thus for instance an elected local politician discussing her relations with representatives of the association of cultural mediators of Trento notes:

> Our situation is that there is an exchange between associations and the local council at the policy ideation stage and then also during the implementation of policies. For example Amic—the association of mediators is an association of migrants and they are first consulted in devising policies and then hired to help with their implementation so as to solve specific problems. (City councilor, Trento, 2006)

There are other examples of successful interventions at the policy ideation stage of both migrant associations and networks of supportive medical personnel, which are generally acting conjunctly as allies. The choice to integrate all migrants in services of a universalistic nature, rather than to create day clinics "devoted" to their specific needs is a choice that has been expressly proposed by pro-migrant associationism and has been accepted and implemented by health institutions in order to avoid an artificial separation or "ghettoization". One can argue the merits and demerits of each approach, but it is important that this deliberation was an open and inclusive process. The choice made, which implies a distinctive ideological position, has reflected a strong mobilization and participation of members of the pro-migrant network. In any event, there are also dedicated services, which whilst being of specific relevance to migrants are available to everybody and are framed as additions to those offered to entire the citizenry. They include for instance services of psychological support for vulnerable users, among which migrants are often over-represented.

Another example of services successfully requested by migrant associations is cultural mediation, which was until recently unavailable in several locations, such as areas of Trento. This service is offered to immigrants by two social cooperatives that collaborate with public institutions (the local branch of the health services, and Cinformi—a municipal institution supporting migrants). It should be noted, however, that the choice to operate through conventions (an ad-hoc legal contract between the public sector and a private organization, including NGOs), implies that the service of mediation is not permanently institutionalized and therefore not structurally integrated in the Provincial Sanitary System. The use of conventions, having a limited temporal duration, creates a strong uncertainty in terms of the continuity of services over time, as they are conditioned by contingent factors, such as budget constraints and changing political will.

The role of civil society is not restricted to organized and carefully planned initiatives. In the Italian context successful changes often take place haphazardly as ad-hoc responses to general problems which, instead of being carefully and globally addressed, are solved by improvised approaches which can then become more permanent. One example concerns the issues of Islamic menus. Here our interviews suggest that when specific requests emerge, solutions are not pursued in general terms trough policy changes but are often ad-hoc.

> We at the local government office have had to face the issue of Islamic menus, but it has proven difficult to approach it in general policy terms. Our food is purchased externally through a tendering process. Our migrant patients are about one percent of all patients and Islamic patients are possibly 0.6%. In this situation we could not justify a tendering process. However, informally patients can ask for a tailored menu, and they do and we accept it as a matter of course. Similarly, the possibility to request a woman doctor for Islamic women has not been legislated upon, but we always satisfy this request. (Local councilor, Naples, 2006)

This flexibility is not only typical of Naples but also occurs in Trento where a similar approach to requests for women doctors is also accepted informally. Health service personnel realize that any request brought to the national level could be used politically by the right. In Trento however, processes of institutional response also take place. For instance it was originally possible for migrant women whose husbands work and whose Italian is not fluent to be allowed to receive visits out of visiting times, for instance in the evening. When this situation recurred for a period, a day-clinic was opened from 6pm to 8pm to meet the needs of the migrant population. However, this initiative has not been labeled as migrant initiative but as a general service to the entire population.

Finally, a more general example of successful contribution of civil society in health-related migrant protection concerns the amelioration of the knowledge base of the medical and administrative personnel. Analysts have noticed that it is frequently still the case that personnel are deeply unaware of the normative aspects of their interaction with migrants; they tend to adopt incorrect procedures, which often result in delays and violations of migrants' rights. The associational network has contributed to making the institutions aware of the problem, pointing to specific breaches, signaling abuses or administrative difficulties. Such problems however have not yet resulted in permanent structural change.

The Role of Civil Society Actors in Implementing Change

In Italy, as in the previous cases, the role of civil society in support of migrants' health needs to be conceptualized in terms of the reactions of the Italian state to migratory trends and the state regulatory traditions reviewed above. More broadly speaking, this role also needs to be framed in terms of organized civil society's efforts to combat the phenomena of xenophobia and racism, which have been frequently identified as prominent in the Italian context. This is a role that has characterized Italian anti-racist movements—a constellation of organizations of different kinds that, in recent years, have increasingly turned to service delivery in various policy sectors on behalf of racially stigmatized citizens.

This support from a conscious constituency of Italian activists is particularly necessary as migrants are characterized by such a high proportion of illegal entries into the country, making them particularly politically disenfranchised and vulnerable users of state services. Coming from a wide range of countries and without reference to the linguistic and cultural features provided by a colonial background compounds this social and political vulnerability. For them, all political activities (ranging from lobbying to public protest activities) are high-risk strategies that can cause expulsion from the country. As they often do not speak the host language, coordinating strategies with allies, sympathetic institutional actors and other social movements remains difficult.

Coordinating activities is difficult even among migrants living in the same area, since they speak many different languages. Since their religions differ, they cannot utilize churches as shared meeting points. They might have different and sometimes incompatible problems, principles and related claims. Finally, they are also often territorially dispersed. Despite discrimination, they find it difficult to mobilize. Their situation epitomizes the 'poor people's movements,' which do not have the political skills, organizing ability and resources to engage in viable political participation (Piven and Cloward 1978).

Migrants in Italy, as in other southern European societies, live and work in much poorer societies than are found in Germany and Canada, and are themselves poorer than many native born citizens. Struggling to find employment often becomes an all-absorbing activity which does not leave time for any form of political participation, contentious or non-contentious. Associations of migrants are also too weak to function as stepping stones for policy effectiveness. They are often merely defensive and culturally-orientated. Nonetheless, a conscious constituency of institutional activists and allies has emerged to oppose racial discrimination, improve quality of life and promote the social recognition and political representation of migrants. It is in this context that Italian civil society supports migrants in the health sector.

Until the early 1990s, pro-migrant Italian civil society could be fairly sharply divided between a Catholic and a left-leaning secular sector. This division has weakened in recent years. The two sectors are now more integrated and they have also become more institutionalized in many respects, directly gaining prominence in local government or in the social economy that is supported by local government.

Civil society volunteers (and to an extent social activists of the new left-liberal movements of the 1980s) have been incorporated into policy-making institutions and have transformed into institutional activists; this also applies to supporters of migrants and their associations. These are often hosted by sectors of leftist parties and other like-minded social organizations (such as trade unions). As part of this process of institutionalization, anti-racist civil society volunteers have been given a consultative role in local councils, thus often merging the service-delivery and the advocacy functions. As a response to the relatively weak Italian state, which is unable to properly deliver services, becoming engaged in service delivery has been seen as a necessity—a logical extension of the ethical imperatives that motivate anti-racist activists, be they Catholic or secular. They then become part of broad anti-racist coalitions, bringing together sectors of leftist parties, third sector organizations, public interest groups (such as civil-rights groups) and service-delivery organizations (such as development NGOs, migrants' associations and some professional or religious organizations). They exert both their advocacy and their service delivery functions in a variety of migrant-related areas, such as health, housing, rehabilitation of drug addicts, support for prostitutes, work with prisoners, cultural initiatives of sensitization of the population, etc.

In this context, the third sector has acquired prominence as an important component of the decision-making system. Both the numerical growth of its organizations and affiliates and their institutionalization redefined and increased its role. Important areas of public policy increasingly rely on the expertise, resources and personnel that this sector provides. As a result, the third sector has come under scrutiny as an interface between the state, the political system and the citizenry. Issues of transparency in the selection of associations and their accountability and effectiveness are at stake. This has implications for pro-migrant associations, as well as for other aspects of civil society. The fact that the national government has been generally controlled by a right-wing coalition in recent years makes the contribution of this sector even more relevant at local level, where many large urban settings with high levels of migrant population are controlled by the center-left. But even in areas where the center-right is in power, local government and the support of the Catholic Church (with its network of parishes) provides effective niches and resources for pro-migrant work in health and other areas.

Although still limited in comparison with other industrialized countries, in Italy (even in its South) this sector has experienced numerical, organizational and thematic expansion, with an organizational growth of over 150 percent in the last ten years and over 21,000 organizations active at present (Testa 2007). As the number of organizations grows faster than the number of people involved, this indicates that increasing thematic diversification and organizational fragmentation is possibly encouraged by the close relationships with other organizations, both politically and service-oriented. In recent years, over 850,000 Italians contributed to the activities of the third sector. Over 12,000 are paid employees, half of whom are paid by the state (Italian National Statistical Institute figures reported in Testa 2007). Over seven million people have benefited from its services, which are provided both by large organizations such as the Catholic ACLI or Caritas and the secular ARCI, as well as by many other small ones. The two large Catholic organizations and the one ex-communist organization constitute the backbone of pro-migrant activities in sectors such as health.

In addition, in Italy, several ex-activists previously engaged in political campaigns took up relevant positions in the third sector in recent years, often forming smaller associations and bringing to the sector an understanding of the importance and techniques of political communication and of politics more generally.

A 2001 study revealed that there were 900 associations operating on behalf of immigrants/ non-Italian citizens in Italy, including 750 promoted by foreign nationals and 150 by Italian activists acting on their behalf (Vicentini and Fava 2001, cited in Caponio 2005). Migrants' own associations were weak, fragmented, small-scale and non- professional, devoting their energies to cultural initiatives rather than political mobilization. They were hardly representative of the migrant population—smaller migrant groups with higher cultural capital formed more associations than larger groups, especially if these were not Catholic and received less help from the Catholic Church. Thus, for instance, there is a higher proportion of Middle Eastern and African associations staffed by students and refugees than there are Chinese associations—a group whose many members are unskilled and whose family-oriented culture hinders associationism (Caponio 2005: 933). The situation has not changed significantly in recent years.

Associations that promote the rights of migrants are then dominated and led by white ethnic Italians, particularly those linked to the trade unions and the Catholic Church. The Catholic association, Caritas, is the most influential and prominent organization working with immigrants, and is highly active both at the national and the local level in organizing a range of social care provisions, including support for health issues.

Caponio's fieldwork on three cities (Naples, Milan and Bologna) suggests that administrations prefer to interact with large, generalist pro-migrant organizations staffed by Italians rather than migrant-run organizations (Caponio 2005; also Caponio 2010). As previously mentioned, this might change, as a second generation of migrants is currently going through the education system and will reach adulthood in a few years. This is particularly the case for the larger migrant communities: people from Albania, Morocco, Romania, China and the Philippines. At the moment, however, several recently formed migrants' associations are not focusing on relations with public administrations. This situation emerges, for instance, in an interview with a CGIL representative from Trento:

> The world of migrant associations is very varied. There are a lot of associations, but they are all very fragile. And I do not speak only of their limited ability to plan actions in defence and for the protection of their rights, but also about their cultural activities. In effect, the only association that has a strong cohesion and a strong presence is the association Iliria, which organizes the Macedonian and the Albanians in the zone of the stone quarries. They have a strong feeling of identity that is born from the fact that they consider themselves a minority oppressed in their homeland. And this leads them to what often appears as exasperated nationalism.. Other migrant associations might occasionally become visible in folkloric contexts, but they not only do not have any ability to be relevant in terms of expressing their needs—they are not even effective in terms of creating community cohesion. (Union representative, Trento, 2006)

Thus, at the moment, large associations and their local branches are the main actors in connecting state structures and pro-migrant efforts, although the number of smaller associations is constantly growing. However, even whilst civil society efforts are constantly growing, the Italian population seems increasingly unwilling to see migrants as legitimate users of state resources, and there are often tensions related to the distribution of welfare state resources.

In addition to these problems related to dominant political discourses and institutional structures, the health needs of migrants are also hindered by distinctive features of the administrative culture of the Italian state. Interviews with Italian civil society personnel and sympathetic civil servants in the health sector suggest that their initiatives on behalf of migrants have been frequently held up by bureaucratic delays, a legalistic approach and a set of dominant cultural assumptions that impinge negatively on the recognition of migrants as a deserving social constituency. The health system is mainly geared to provide services of a very specialized nature, and consequently the user is first and foremost conceptualized as a subject in need of health services, not as a social carrier of identities, including religious, ethnic and racial ones. This is often problematic for migrants, as their needs often cross the boundary between specific health needs and needs more generally related to their social, religious, linguistic or cultural identities, which can easily be conceptualized as not pertinent (i.e., not being part of the dominant narrow definition of the remit of health services). These needs then seem less urgent and less central to the duties and expectations of health services. This situation is compounded by the fact that these broader categories of needs are often not clearly expressed by migrants. One then sees a general willingness to listen to all claims from users, but to the extent that in the Italian context of still new and uprooted migrants specific claims are often not advanced with reference to minority identities, they are not conceptualized as distinctive and important. Consequently, they are not acted upon.

Agents of Change: Health Care Professionals and Migrant Representatives

Data from interviews in Germany, Canada and Italy reveals that a few key factors shape how the stakeholders discuss and initiate institutional reforms, and to what extent access to health services is enhanced from these efforts. Two main factors are whether there are cultural mediators (also called translators in the German case) in the system and whether there is staff from the minority or migrant community. Another key factor is the availability of institutional actors with a strong pro-migrant ethical commitment—these are for instance doctors, but also local political actors, prominent members of the clergy and high-level civil servants. These institutional actors have sometimes been named "institutional activists" to indicate the processes whereby through their agency institutional resources and legitimacy are utilized on behalf of a political cause—in this case a principled support for migrants as a vulnerable constituency (for the concept of "institutional activist," see Santoro and McGuire 1997). In the following paragraphs we will consider these aspects in more detail. We will show that hiring staff with a migration background is intentionally pursued in Canada and is sometimes the unintentional result of job market dynamics in Italy, whilst the strategy of providing mediators tends to be the dominant one in Germany and Italy. Finally, in Italy the role of institutional activists will play a distinctive role. However, even within these broad approaches there are marked differences among the cases we examined.

Comparing the cases of Germany and Canada reveals three patterns in terms of approaches to incorporating translators, cultural mediators and staff from culturally diverse backgrounds. In both cases there is a consensus on the significance of the language barriers in accessing services. Accordingly there are initiatives in both Germany and Canada to overcome this challenge. However the main difference between the two cases is that in Germany the practice of incorporating and training translators and cultural mediators is more ad hoc and informal while in Canada in both provinces there are formal attempts, institutions and structures. Nevertheless even in Canada there is a discrepancy in terms of the use of the services formally provided and the structure of the formal training. This difference is observed not only across provinces but also within the same province among different hospitals in the same city. Second, in Germany there is some disagreement among the health care professionals whether distinct services are needed for cultural communities at all. In Canada there is no indication of such contention among health care professionals. Third, both systems view the role of cultural mediators as even more important than the translators alone. Both systems also emphasize the significance of having translators and cultural mediators understand health matters to complement their language skills. Fourth, in both systems costs concerning the use of services seem to be a major determinant of how frequently the formal services are used. Relying on culturally diverse hospital staff appears as a much more convenient solution for health care professionals and policy practitioners in both countries while acknowledging the risks involved in such band-aid solution approach. Fifth, training of health care professionals themselves is seen as also pivotal in building a system whereby the health professionals are equipped with culturally sensitive training before they begin practicing medicine.

Strategies to overcome challenges in providing advocacy and delivering health services to migrant groups differ in Germany, Canada and Italy. In Canada, there is a more macro-level institutional problem solving strategy whereby institutional solutions are pursued through introducing multicultural programs to existing health service delivery or promoting initiatives targeting these communities directly, often in collaboration with community associations. In Germany the focus is more on the micro-level aiming to promote employment of staff from diverse communities to advance multicultural health service delivery in the system. In Italy, there are different strategies between the two case studies of Trento and Naples. In Trento a concerted effort to support migrants in integrated ways is exerted by generalist Catholic associationism working together with local institutions. They typically conceptualize migrants as vulnerable users of all public services and therefore seek to support them across a broad range of needs. This perspective, we will argue, is an expression of the social Catholicism that has historically characterized the political culture and the civil society of Trento. Conversely, in Naples institutions partially replace a weak or inexistent civil society. These substantially different approaches require a more detailed examination.

In Germany the debate about promoting migrant specific health care mostly revolves around whether or not and how to employ hospital staff with culturally diverse backgrounds. In Montreal and Vancouver there is a clear emphasis on community health partnerships rather than focusing solely on employment of staff from diverse cultural backgrounds. This is partly a result of the policy framework providing room for multiculturalism in the health care system and partly a consequence of having to rely on fewer financial resources in hospitals. Then the health care system turns to the community groups and volunteer associations for supporting the needs of diverse communities.

It is suggested that programs such as health promotion initiatives to raise awareness, can be more effectively delivered through community groups, so there are cases where there has been a transfer of resources and responsibilities to community associations to operate these programs. Many of the initiatives promoted by civil society actors are primarily through collaboration between community associations and health services organizations. In addition, there are a variety of advocacy strategies adopted by community groups to raise awareness about the issues of diversity, and to inform community groups about the availability of services.

Conclusions: Strategies of Change in the Heath Care Sector

As previously pointed out, the structural features of the unorganized and organized civil societies of the different countries we analyzed shape their modes of operation and strategies in supporting migrants in the health field. On the basis of these constraints, civil society can play a multiplicity of roles, which range from providing information to policy-makers to representing minorities in the national and local political process, to improving service delivery in a targeted fashion. All of these factors in the health field can be condensed into two main overarching roles: improving access to the system and improving the system's response to migrants' needs both in terms of advocacy and at the stage of service delivery. We have reviewed efforts to improve access in the previous chapter. In this chapter, we have discussed issues of advocacy and service delivery in the three case studies. In the concluding section, we will now discuss what general patterns emerge and what lessons can be learned in terms of strategies to improve migrant-friendly services.

Considering the three cases contextually reveals a set of related issues. First, the universalism of health entitlements is a principle that can be used instrumentally to avoid questioning actual inequalities. This has emerged consistently in interviews in the German case. For instance, as mentioned in an interview, a Bremen integration officer argued that promoting an intercultural aperture of the system was unnecessary given the principle of universalism, which should dispense policy-makers of the need for additional efforts. A similar situation emerges in Italy, where the state is seen as ideally above particularistic interests. In this context and in the context of a population with sizeable sectors hostile to migrants (Ruzza and Fella 2011; Saint-Blancat and Friedberg 2005), the right to health tends to be mainly accepted as a right to general provisions of public services. Migrant-specific services are then sometimes framed by center-right parties as "special-favours."

Thus, in all contexts, whilst a universalist ethos is accepted in principle, efforts to guarantee the implementation of universal access meets with structured variation that denies such access in practice. However, reactions to this denial of services are argued differently in the different countries according to their respective political cultures. Thus, given the Italian political myth of an impartial Napoleonic state, it is then not a coincidence that migrant associations prefer to frame their demands for migrant-specific services as provisions that can benefit the entire population and be presented as universal services. This instrumental and restricting use of the universalist ethos is less pronounced in Canada, where multiculturalist provisions and a multiculturalist ethos are well entrenched in the system.

Secondly, institutional mechanisms are important and changes in the way they operate can have unforeseen and relevant consequences. Two competing principles are clashing and shaping the provision of services in distinctive ways. On the one hand, there are often paradigmatic changes in the way health is administered and this has a decisive impact on the population. Thus, for instance, after changes in the supervision of health care provision were made in Germany and politicians acquired direct representation on hospital governing boards, the delayed impact of the population's hostility to aspects of multiculturalism had a negative impact on the aperture of the system. As a consequence of this change the regional government has virtually lost its political influence in the hospital, particularly in reference to the legal framework defining its *modus operandi*, and is solely involved in the hospital planning committee. Thus, instead of institutionalized migrant-friendly policies, one can now observe the impact of the vagaries of public opinion on political actors.

More broadly, paradigmatic changes such as this one reveal a fundamental uncertainty with regard to issues of accountability and transparency in the way public services are organized—an uncertainty that has marked the entire sector of public service provision in Western countries, where considerations of efficiency, cost-effectiveness and even representativeness have clashed and pushed the systems sometimes in the direction of more technical and managerial restructuring along principles of *New Public Management*. In other cases, a more prominent role for political actors as guarantors of representativeness has emerged, as illustrated in the previously mentioned German case. In addition, paradigmatic changes occur more frequently in the case of migration because of its direct political salience for party politics. Thus, changes of coalitions often mean a major disjuncture in the way services are organized. We see this for instance in the Italian case, where the center-right coalition has frequently attempted and sometimes successfully managed to restrict the previously universalist ethos by requiring doctors to report illegal migrants that access services.

However, in addition to occasional but disruptive paradigmatic change, the health systems also appear in a constant state of low-level flux where path-dependent dynamics over time radically alter the working of several institutional structures. A positive example of path dependency is the Canadian liaison workers project aimed at providing workers who can accompany the patient throughout the health care system. This project transformed from its initial focus on the facilitation of appropriate service use to a partnership with the immigrant settlement services organizations. A similar gradual expansion of activities has also been evident in the Italian case of the SIMM, which has expanded its network, relations with policy-makers and a range of initiatives over time. While adjustments to the institutional framework are natural and necessary in any policy domain, the fact that they tend to occur so frequently in the Italian case seems to indicate that policy approaches are still not stable.

Frequent changes reveal an overall lack of institutionalization of the systems, which is partly dependent on the irregularity of migration fluxes, the continuing political salience of the migration issue and its use in electoral competition, as well as the constantly changing social features and needs of the migrant population. With regard to both paradigmatic and path-dependent readjustments, our research has pointed out the need for resiliency within the health system—a need which is often difficult to address.

Institutional innovation is not only spurred by political and macroeconomic dynamics or by path-dependencies. A sizeable amount of innovation is also emerging out of improvised contingent arrangements. This is particularly an aspect of the Italian case, with its frequent reliance on *ad-hoc* solutions, which are then presented and labeled as addressing the general needs of the population, rather than as targeting a migrant base. Innovations promoted in this way, such as after-hour service provisions or the possibility of after-hour visits to patients, become then at times institutionalized.

In addition to these general traits, however, there are also relevant differences of philosophy and state capacity that are revealed by the way the different systems operate, their priorities, and how institutional reform takes place. In Germany, the system mostly focuses on language translation and hiring immigrant staff. However, as in Italy, the high level of politicization of the migrant issue results in a continuing contention over whether migrant-friendly services should be provided. In Italy, the issue of migrants' health activates a widespread, but not always effective mobilization of generalist civil society organizations and a related strong reliance on the intermediation of Italian associations in both service delivery and advocacy functions. Generalist civil society associations are also assuming a growing role in enabling migrants' associations to develop independent policy and service delivery skills. However, this takes place in a general context of mounting negative attitudes toward migrants and their problems. In this way, the Italian model is more similar to the German case than to the Canadian case. In Canada, there is clearly a higher commitment to multiculturalism at all levels of governance and a strong impact of a federalized structure of the state, which enables provincial initiatives that address challenges of diversity and partnerships with the community.

Despite different emphases on the merits of federalist arrangements, actual territorial variability is not, however, a uniquely Canadian characteristic. Our research revealed a patchwork of initiatives, which are often as varied within states as they are between them. Differences are prominent not only at the local level, but also at the regional level in both Germany and Italy. Furthermore, this difference is growing, as a gradual process of regionalization has marked Europe since the 1970s and is now accelerating in several respects. Particularly in Italy, a federalist reform of the state is under way, which involves relevant changes in the health sector. Health care in Canada has also gone through a process of regionalization similar to that seen in Italy.

A second set of lessons we can learn from these cases concerns the factors that drive developments of the policy agenda and areas in which new initiatives have proven successful. In Canada, successful initiatives included promoting cultural mediators and activating community involvement, through the use of health facilitators and diversity coordinators to both facilitate immigrants' knowledge of health care, and in addressing the need to train hospital staff. In Germany, successful initiatives develop mostly in relation to translation and to some extent following efforts to hire more culturally diverse staff in the health system. In Italy, the pro-migrant agenda is typically driven by Italian professionals and generalist third sector personnel. Initiatives that involve prestigious professionals, such as doctors working on the behalf of migrants, have been particularly successful. As previously mentioned, in a fundamentally hierarchical and corporatist society, the role of medical experts has proven essential not only in interfacing with state authorities, but also in liaising with health authorities of migrants' countries of origin.

Finally, in considering the three case studies contextually, one realizes how the policy agenda is in part determined by the actual needs of the migrant population; however, equally important is how different systems come to conceptualize social and political problems given their unique political cultures. Here, one could identify "garbage can" dynamics whereby favorite solutions are made applicable to an almost unrelated set of problems—a dynamic that not coincidentally has been identified in other areas of migration policy (Cohen et al. 1972; Guiraudon 2003). In this context, the Canadian normative entrenchment of multiculturalism and the acknowledgement of the value of diversity at all levels of governance leads to the focus on health systems' ability to respond to the needs of diverse populations. Conversely, in the Italian context, the strong tradition of social Catholicism defines migrants' needs in terms of a continuation of provisions for support and care of the needy poor. The social controversy that then typically emerges in reaction to this framing is between a center-right that attempts to redefine migrants as the undeserving poor, justifying the limitation of access and services on this basis, and a center-left which opposes it. When this controversy takes place, which is also to an extent the case in Germany, the policy machinery may just stall and produce *ad-hoc* solutions. Typically, in Germany, one finds a deficient legal framework that is unable to satisfactorily promote intercultural initiatives and an abundance of *ad-hoc* and informal efforts which are often isolated and unable to become properly institutionalized.

Conclusion: Political Advocacy and Institutional Change in the Health Care System

A Changing Political Opportunity Structure

Health care provision is governed by more than the simple organizational task of providing effective services for citizens in need of medical treatment. Whilst it is administered by distinct organizational imperatives and institutional rules,[1] it is also a contested arena of public policy: The scope and form of this essential public service is a matter of politically controversial debate. Issues of access, quality of care and distribution of intrinsically scarce resources are subject to continuous contestation. What is apparent in the three national contexts under investigation in our study is that this struggle over the proper organization of health care provision is critically guided by discursive representations of what is appropriate, just and legitimate. As Jane Jenson described it succinctly: "The terrain on which actors struggle for representation is the universe of political discourse, a space in which socially-constructed … practices and meaning systems jostle with each other for social attention and legitimacy" (Jenson 1989: 237–38). Health care is also such a discursive terrain upon which marginalized and less-privileged groups and their representatives seek attention, articulate their needs and try to promote institutional reforms. The discursive representation structures the perspective of key actors and opens or closes institutional venues for change. In this respect, it depicts the legitimacy and authority of claims made by actors who speak on behalf of migrants and minorities.

The task of accommodating cultural diversity is an issue that has proven to be a considerable challenge to the health care systems in Canada, Germany, and Italy. There is ample evidence that migrants are less likely than other citizens to access health care services and that the chronic underutilization of services can also be interpreted as an issue of failed intercultural aperture on the institutional level. At a high level of generalization, one can speak about a relatively low degree of institutional openness in spite of the manifest underutilization of services and problems of access experienced by particular groups of migrants and

1 From the perspective of organizational sociology, one could argue that the health care sector follows a systemic *modus operandum* that, with its commitment to universal access, is relatively adverse to political reform driven by the multiculturalist agenda.

minorities. Unlike other areas of public life (such as, for instance, the field of education), demands for more sensitivity for and responsiveness to the challenge of accommodating cultural diversity have been rather tame. Beyond issues of institutional inertia and the difficult task of introducing operative changes in highly complex organizational systems, there is a forceful concern about the potential risk involved in allowing for culturally-sensitive and group-specific entitlements in the provision of health care. Our interviews in Germany and Italy—and to lesser degree also in Canada—show a robust and principled orientation toward a universalistic ethos. The main challenge of state-governed health care systems has historically been and often still is to provide comprehensive coverage to all citizens and to overcome the exclusion of marginalized groups. One could speak of a kind of political-culturalist path-dependency governed by the rationale of inclusiveness *vis-à-vis* the economically deprived and strong reservations regarding group-differentiated approaches. We detected this discursive representation of health care within the normative universe of distributive justice and universal access to be particularly strong among those working in the health care sector and political representatives from the moderate left.

Yet, this discursive representation of health plays out differently in the political arenas and policy deliberations in the three national contexts that we investigated. In our European case studies, for instance, we observed how the recent backlash against multiculturalism (Schain 2006; Sniderman et al. 2006; Vertovec and Wessendorf 2009) has changed the political opportunity structure for launching initiatives to accommodate cultural diversity in the health care sector. Next to the concern about compromising the integrity of universally accessible health care, our interviewees from Germany and Italy often describe the claims of migrants and minorities as illegitimate and a genuine threat to liberal democracies. The discursive opportunity structure for advancing responses to cultural diversity is thus shaped by strong reservations from the Left and the Right alike: While the social democratic Left in Europe has demonstrated lukewarm responses to an agenda that seems to be antagonistic to its core principle of redistributive justice, the Right has increasingly endorsed a more aggressive anti-multicultural stance, portraying the issue of accommodating cultural diversity as threat to, rather than a desirable corrective for individually-based liberal democracy.

In the Canadian context, such a highly antagonistic political environment in which the health care system is confronted with the challenge of cultural diversity does not exist like in the German or Italian context. With the legacy of over 40 years of multiculturalism as state policy, approaches to dealing with cultural diversity are far more guided by pragmatic concerns for incremental reform than the general debate about the alleged conflict between general norms of equality versus group-specific rights and entitlements. Our study leads us to assume that this de-dramatization of identity conflicts has also to do with the way in which multiculturalism in Canada has opened institutional channels for migrants and minorities to articulate their needs and to become outspoken actors in the public debate on the legitimate status of group rights in society. Somewhat counterintuitive and contrary to the popular assumption about the link between cultural diversity and political radicalization, in our interviews from Canada there is hardly any concern about the potential threat that migrant and minority organizations might pose to public life and principles of individual rights-based liberalism. Rather, the actual experiences of urban centers with a high density of ethno-cultural minorities seem to indicate that the inclusion of these groups into public-political life has at least opened the possibility of a gradual institutional learning process in the health care sector. While there is always the danger of mere symbolic consultation in the political process for legitimating purposes, political inclusion of minority groups and institutional innovation can set into motion a mutually reinforcing dynamic that results in notable effects on policy formation.

Locality matters in how processes of advocacy and institutional reform unfold; however, it is not only the national context that determines them. Our comparative analysis highlighted that locality significantly matters when it comes to migrants' role in the policy-process and, related to this, changes in the health care system. Specifically, sub-national levels of governance have developed into meaningful arenas of political debate and policy formation. Irrespective of national policies, some cities shared more similarities with respect to migrants' access to health care than cities within the same national territory. This casts doubt upon the legal system as a main determinant of local access structures and confirms recent findings on the growing significance of territorial levels of governance as arenas for public deliberation (Glick Schiller and Caglar 2009, 2011).

The Form, Scope and Effects of Political Advocacy in the Health Care System

The broader political context shapes opportunities for action and openings for institutional reforms. However, it does not determine the form in which migrants advocate their interests and what effect these efforts have on the operation of the health care system. Our three national and six local contexts allowed us to shed light on the considerable variation in terms of action strategies, actor coalitions and responses in the health care sector. At times our interviews seemed to suggest that much depends on distinct constellations on the ground, determined individuals in the health care system or culturally-sensitive projects that grow out of idiosyncratic circumstances in particular institutional settings. Still, there are some generalizable patterns that our six-city study allows us to detect in the interplay between migrant and pro-migrant associations, health care authorities and policy-makers. We identified the following key variables in this respect.

Strength and Degree of Organization of Migrant Community

The numerical concentration of migrant communities is a critical factor with respect to their ability to gain a voice and access to public deliberation and policy processes: Well-established and resourceful migrant communities are likely to have a whole array of opportunities at their disposal to make their concerns heard and intervene politically. Over time, migrant communities develop organizational resources, networks of advocacy and (in)formal modes of engaging political authorities. Manifestly urban centers are the central arena in which these political struggles for influence play out. It is in bigger and more prosperous cities, with their locally distinct social and political opportunities, where migrant and minority associations find the resources and resonance for promoting the interests of their respective constituencies.

Vancouver and Montreal are examples of well-established migrant communities with a long legacy of organizational representation and network-building. Advocacy in the health care sector can rely on these entrenched modes of engaging the public and policy community. In Italian cities, contrastingly, these migrant communities are a relatively recent phenomenon. Often, these groups do not reach a critical threshold in terms of their numerical strength, nor can they rely on a repertoire of political intervention that develops with experience and networking over time. The situation is similar in Leipzig: It is only with German unification some 20 years ago that a significant group of migrants started to settle in this city and were no longer prevented from interacting with the receiving society, leaving this community without an infrastructure to rely upon. Besides, the migrant ratio in Leipzig nevertheless remained relatively low as compared to many West German cities.

In contrast, Bremen is a city with a well-established migrant community. However, this community's political intervention abilities have been restricted due to severe funding cuts in recent years. Migrant and minority organizations often depend on some form of funding and state authorities play a critical role in allowing them to operate in an effective fashion. In the Canadian context, many of the actors that have become spokespersons for migrant communities could rely on a relatively well-funded infrastructure for migrant associations also in their capacity as service providers (often as part of the settlement industry) and thus on the essential organizational resources to raise concerns, represent their constituency or launch campaigns. In the Italian context, the relatively small and young migrant communities often are dependent on the organizational capacities and networks of established, mainstream civil society actors. While this proves to be an effective way to compensate for their lack of organizational resources, this strategy has important repercussions on how and through which channels political advocacy is feasible.

Degree of Openness of Policy Process

The receptiveness of the political addressee to political claims is apparently of immediate relevance for the form and effects of migrants' political advocacy. Even if, as in Montreal and Vancouver, the partial inclusion of migrant organizations into the policy process does not give them significant authority in the decision-making process, this position has empowering effects. It provides civil society groups with direct access to political authorities, even if they are in a position to neglect the expertise and concerns of these groups. Political advocacy becomes more effective if migrant associations are considered a genuine part of public deliberations and if community engagement over health issues has become a routinized procedure for legitimizing policy decisions. The long-term effects of such access to the policy process can also be measured in terms of indirectly influencing key decisions by providing information and setting the agenda. Establishing non-state representatives of migrants as legitimate and accepted spokespersons for the community makes it increasingly difficult to simply neglect them when their interests in the health system are concerned. It is under these conditions that migrant associations can establish themselves as important nodes in the policy process, where their expertise becomes an indispensable asset for acquiring information and legitimacy.

In contrast, in our German and Italian case studies, civil society advocacy groups are almost entirely excluded from the policy process. Much of their effort is unavoidably directed at circumventing established modes of public deliberation and decision-making. In addition, in the face of their low socioeconomic status, combined with decreasing legitimacy and resources, many migrants seem to abandon associational forms as an avenue of claim-making. The situation is similar in Italy, where the current conservative government has closed many consultative institutions and embraced an anti-multiculturalist ethos that does not facilitate efforts at establishing a viable presence of migrant organizations in civil society. In turn, the Italian Left has been an articulate and political advocate for migrants' and minorities' rights. However, this form of political advocacy is very much based on established church or civil society-based organizations in which migrants themselves only play a very marginal role.

Ability to Build Cross-Sectoral Coalitions

One critical factor with respect to successful attempts of civil society actors advocating for migrant-friendly services is the ability to build coalitions among migrant associations, political authorities and health care representatives. Where representatives from these contexts are engaged in meaningful deliberation it is most likely, as many of our examples of institutional reform illustrate, that the claims of migrants and minorities are considered seriously and trigger change. In particular, when management-level professionals from the health sector are willing to participate in such fora of exchange, it becomes feasible to overcome the deeply ingrained fear of outside interference.

This becomes particularly relevant once health care workers themselves become active and play an influential role in this process. We found that front-line health workers (even more so than the hospital management) can take on a critical bridging function. Their intimate knowledge of internal procedure can foster a kind of "compatibility" between the demands of civil society associations and those working within the health care sector. They can translate concerns about cultural diversity and appropriate care into day-to-day organizational practices.

Health care workers can also become important initiators of institutional change, often acting in two overlapping roles: as representatives of civil society groups and as professionals in the health care system. In Germany, change was often created by concerned medical staff (with and without a migration background) who were confronted with migrants' access barriers. In particular, the second generation of migrants who work in the health system, be it as care providers or in managerial positions, have made notable institutionalized efforts to improve care for migrants and non-migrants with low socio-economic status. This indicates that increasing levels of second generation migrant education is positively related to migrant activism, claim-making and, as a result, the lowering of access barriers in the health care system.

However, what is often being compromised in grassroots' pushes for institutional change is the scope and sustainability of what can be achieved in terms of services and regulations that reflect migrants' needs. Given how change is advocated here, we often find distinctly local initiatives for the improvement of service delivery. Indeed, health care workers often have only limited interaction with and support from broader advocacy groups or political authorities. Their attempts to introduce migrant-friendly services and routines in their daily work are often shaped by their immediate work environment and, as a result, are limited in scope. This might be an important reason as to why we found such a surprising variation with respect to provision of services in the health care system that are sensitive to the needs of the migrant population. The availability of such services for migrants and minorities varies even across individual cities and regularly reflects locally distinct constellations of actors (very prominently, concerned health care professional).

At the same time, we found that such small-scale and limited local initiatives can trigger a momentous institutional learning process. While health care organizations prove to be relatively adverse to outside pressure, they tend to respond well to operational changes that come from within and that are organizationally compatible with the procedural norms of institutional routines. In this respect, even small-scale initiatives can trigger considerable institutional change through imitation and learning processes. Then again, this depends on there being channels of communication and distribution in place in order to spread the knowledge about best practices.

Resonance with Functional Imperatives of the Health Care System

Political advocacy and suggestions for institutional reform were most likely to be successful if they resonated with the functional imperatives of the health care system. While the cultural aperture is often perceived to be a normatively questionable and organizationally difficult proposition for change, arguments that effectively link issues of cultural diversity with those of immediate relevance for optimizing health care provision are prone to instigate change. Campaigns relating cultural diversity to reducing patients' risks and the quality of care are particularly likely to be picked up by health care professionals or policy-makers. Similarly, considerations of cost reduction and efficient use of scarce resources in the health care system can have enabling effects if culturally-sensitive services are advocated for in terms of cost-saving measures[2] and optimizing procedural efficiencies.

Another important aspect in this respect is how the claims of migrants and minorities are "decoded" by representatives in the health care system. What resurfaced in our interviews, in Germany and Italy in particular, was how their claims are rejected when their diversity is grounded in religious or cultural terms, but not when they are conceptualized as users of state services with special needs. In the latter case, the health care system can classify them just as any other public-interest group that demands better treatment and more appropriate services. In this context, their advocacy and special needs are conceived as legitimate because they address a *de facto* inequality of rights of a particular segment of the population. Yet, once this particularistic interest is introduced into the policy area in terms of a defense of intrinsic cultural or religious differences, it is likely to lose this legitimacy. The frame of reference thus tends to no longer be the pluralist struggle for specific group interests in the health sector; rather, it becomes a (potentially threatening) issue of identity (particularly religious ones, such as a Muslim identity).

Again, promoting institutional reform in the health care sector is fundamentally dependent on a successful framing strategy: In the health care system, goals of cultural aperture or group-specific services are often perceived as too difficult to address and disruptive in their practical implications. Yet, framing the issue in terms of improving essential aspects of service provision beyond the group of migrants and as part of a free market economy that builds on increasing "customers" proves to be instrumental in overcoming institutional inertia. It is when the multiculturalist ethos is framed in conjunction with functional imperatives under which the health care system operates that new services are considered and, at times, implemented.

Our transatlantic comparison suggests that there is a demonstrable link between productive institutional solutions in the health care system and the degree to which those affected by it (in our case, migrants and minorities as well as their organized representatives) become part of the decision-making process. This does not mean that complex systems such as health care change from one day to the other in response to the articulated needs of groups without proper access. The process unfolds as a lengthy and often tiresome deliberative process, exchange of ideas and efforts at collaboration. Still, it is this community-based

2 In Germany pro-migrant advocates argue that migrant-friendly structures lead to cost reduction. However, so far no research has proven this causal link and only few hospitals, mainly private ones, have based their structural changes toward more migrant-friendly services on this consideration.

cross-sectoral form of deliberation that proved instrumental in promoting institutional reforms in the health sector.

This raises the issue of creating fora for civil society inclusion and providing them with a meaningful place in the formation and reform of public policies such as health care. Political engagement that lives up to the expectations of community stakeholders from a grassroots perspective is critically dependent on a sustainable process of trust-building among stakeholders in the community and on providing them with the necessary organizational resources to become involved. However, the beneficial effect would not only be the empowering of a marginalized group that formerly had no voice in the decision-making process. Positive outcomes could also be expected for the health care sector itself: The inclusion of stakeholders in the deliberation process promises to lead to more informed decisions and better outcomes. Giving migrants, minorities and other marginalized groups a voice in the system is prone to improve health care delivery and societal inclusion of newcomers more generally. Providing venues and institutional settings for making such outreach and consultation a routine practice would thus be a promising path toward an effective and desirable public policy.

Bibliography

Abu-Laban, Y. and Gabriel, C. 2002. *Selling Diversity. Immigration, Multiculturalism, Employment Equity, and Globalization*. Peterborough: Broadview Press.

Abu-Laban, Y. and Nieguth, T. 2000. Reconsidering the constitution, ethnic minorities, and politics in Canada. *The Canadian Journal of Political Science*, 33(3), 465–97.

Adamson, J. et al. 2003. Ethnicity, socio-economic position and gender – do they affect reported health-care seeking behaviour? *Social Science and Medicine*, 57, 895–904.

Ager, A. and Strang, A. 2008. Understanding integration, a conceptual framework. *Journal of Refugee Studies*, 21(2), 166–91.

Alba, R. and Nee, V. 2003. *Remaking the American Mainstream, Assimilation and Contemporary Immigration*. Cambridge, MA. Harvard University Press.

Ali, J.S., McDermott, S. and Gravel, R.G. 2004. Recent research on immigrant health form statistics Canada's population surveys. *Canadian Journal of Public Health-Revue Canadienne De Sante Publique*, 953, 91–113.

Allasino E., Baptiste F. and Bulsei G.L. 1995. Gli incerti confini, politiche per gli immigrati e politiche di lotta all'esclusione sociale a Torino e Lione. *Polis*, IX(1), 23–44.

Anheier, H. 2009. What kind of nonprofit Sector, what kind of society? Comparative policy reflections. *American Behavioral Scientist*, 52(7), 1082–94.

Asanin, J. and Wilson, K. 2008. "I spent nine years looking for a doctor," Exploring access to health care among immigrants in Mississauga, Ontario, Canada. *Social Science & Medicine*, 666, 1271–83.

Asher, C. and Sciortino, G. 2004. Italian immigration, the origins, nature and evolution of Italy's migratory systems. *Journal of Modern Italian Studies*, 9(1), 49–70.

Bader, V.M. 1998. Egalitarian multiculturalism, institutional separation and cultural pluralism, in *Blurred Boundaries*, edited by R. Bauböck and J. Rundell. Aldershot: Ashgate, 185–222.

Bahadir, S. 2011. *Dolmetschinszenierungen: Kulturen, Identitäten, Akteure*. Berlin: Saxa Verlag.

Barry, B. 1991. Political accommodation and consociational democracy, in *Democracy and Power: Essays in Political Theory 1*, edited by B. Barry. Oxford: Clarendon Press, 100–35.

Barry, B. 1995. *Justice as Impartiality*. Oxford: Clarendon Press.

Barry, B. 2002. *Culture and Equality, An Egalitarian Critique of Multiculturalism*. Cambridge: Harvard University Press.

Barth, F. (ed.) 1969. *Ethnic Groups and Boundaries. The Social Organization of Cultural Difference*. Boston: Little, Brown.

Bauböck, R. 1996. Social and cultural integration in civil society, in *The Challenge of Diversity, Integration and Pluralism in Societies of Immigration*, edited by R. Bauböck, A. Heller and A.R. Zolberg. Aldershot: Ashgate, 67–132.

Bauböck, R. 2002a. Political community beyond the sovereign state. Supranational federalism and transnational minorities, in *Conceiving Cosmopolitanism, Theory, Context and Practice*, edited by S. Vertovec and R. Cohen. Oxford: Oxford University Press, 110–36.

Bauböck, R. 2002b. Farewell to multiculturalism? Sharing values and identities in societies of immigration. *Journal of International Migration and Integration*, 3(1), 1–18.

Bauböck, R. 2003. Reinventing urban citizenship. *Citizenship Studies*, 7(2), 139–59.

Baumann, G. 1996. *Contesting Culture*. Cambridge: Cambridge University Press.

Baumann, G. 1999. *The Multicultural Riddle. Rethinking National, Ethnic and Religious Identities*. New York and London: Routledge.

Baumann, G., Kastoryano, R., Schiffauer, W. and Vertovec, S. (eds) 2002. *Staat – Schule – Ethnizität. Politische Intergration von Immigrantenkindern in vier europäischen Ländern*. Münster/New York/Munich/Berlin: Waxmann.

Baumann, G., Vertovec, S., Schiffauer, W. and Kastoryano, R. (eds) 2004. *Civil Enculturation: Nation-State, School and Ethnic Difference in the Netherlands, Britain, Germany and France*. New York: Berghahn.

Beiser, M. 2005. The health of immigrants and refugees in Canada. *Canadian Journal of Public Health-Revue Canadienne De Sante Publique*, 96(2), 30–44.

Beiser, M. and Stewart, M. 2005. Reducing health disparities – A priority for Canada. *Canadian Journal of Public Health-Revue Canadienne De Sante Publique*, 96(2), 4–5.

Benhabib, S. 2002. *The Claims of Culture. Equality and Diversity in the Global Era*. Princeton, NJ: Princeton University Press.

Berger, M., Galonska, C. and Koopmans, R. 2004. Political integration by a detour? Ethnic communities and social capital of migrants in Berlin. *Journal of Ethnic and Migration Studies*, 30, 491–517.

Berthet, T. and Poirier, C. 2000. Politiques locales d'intégration et immigrants aisés, une comparaison France Québec. *Politique et sociétés*, 19(2–3), 181–213.

Bevelander, P. and Pendakur, R. 2009. Social capital and voting participation of immigrants and minorities in Canada. *Ethnic and Racial Studies*, 328, 1406–30.

Bigot, G. and Fella, S. 2008. The Prodi government's proposed citizenship reform, and the debate on immigration and its impact in Italy. *Modern Italy*, 13(3), 305–15.

Bloemraad, I. 2002. The North American naturalization gap. An institutional approach to citizenship acquisition in the United States and Canada. *International Migration Review*, 36(1), 193–228.

Bommes, M. 2007. Kommunen und nachholende Integrationspolitik – Handlungsperspektiven und Handlungsspielräume, in *Nachholende Integrationspolitik und Gestaltungsperspektiven der Integrationspraxis*, edited by K.J. Bade and H.-G. Hiesserich, Göttingen: V&R unipress, 97–113.

Bommes, M. and Geddes, A. (eds) 2000. *Immigration and Welfare. Challenging the Borders of the Welfare State*. London: Routledge.

Bommes, M. and Thränhardt, D. (eds) 2010. *National Paradigms of Migration Research*. (IMIS-Schriften), Göttingen: V&R unipress.

Borkert, M., Bosswick, W., Heckmann, F. and Lüken-Klaβen. 2007. *Local Integration Policies for Migrants in Europe*. Luxembourg: European Foundation for the Improvement of Living and Working Conditions; European Commission.

Bousetta, H. 2000. Institutional theories of immigrant ethnic mobilisation, relevance and limitation. *Journal of Ethnic and Migration Studies*, Special Issue, 25, 229–45.

Bousetta, H. 2001. *Post-Immigration Politics and the Political Mobilisation of Ethnic Minorities. A Comparative Case Study of Moroccans in Four European Cities*, paper presented at the ECPR Joint Sessions, Grenoble.

Bowl, R. 2007. The need for change in UK mental health services, South Asian service users' views. *Ethnicity & Health*, 121, 1–19.

Bozzini, E. and Fella, S. 2008. The role of civil society in immigration policy making in Italy, changing patterns of conflictual cooperation. *Policy & Politics*, 36(2), 245–59.

Bradford, N. 2004. Place matters and multi-level governance, perspectives on a new urban policy paradigm. *Policy Options*, 25(2), 39–45.

Brenner, N. 1999. Beyond state-centrism? Space, territoriality, and geographical scale in globalization studies. *Theory and Society*, 28, 39–78.

Caponio, T. 2005. Policy networks and immigrants' associations in Italy, The cases of Milan, Bologna and Naples. *Journal of Ethnic and Migration Studies*, 31, 931–50.

Caponio, T. 2008. Immigration research in Italy. A European comparative perspective. *The Sociological Quarterly*, 49(3), 445–64.

Cairns, A.C. et al. (eds) (1999). *Citizenship, Diversity and Pluralism*. Montreal and Kingston: McGill-Queen's University Press.

Carens, J. 2000. *Culture, Citizenship, and Community*. Oxford: Oxford University Press.

Carley, M., Chapman, M., Hastings, A., Kirk, K. and Young, R. 2000. *Urban Regeneration through Partnership, a Critical Appraisal*. Available at: www.jrf.org.uk/knowledge/findings/foundations/560.asp [accessed 26 June 2010].

Castles, S. and Miller, M. 2003. *The Age of Migration, International Population Movements in the Modern World* (3rd edition). Basingstoke: Palgrave Macmillan.

Chambers, S. and Kymlicka, W. (eds) 2002. *Alternative Conceptions of Civil Society*. Princeton: Princeton Unniversity Press.

Cheong, P.H., Edwards, R., Gouldbourne, H. and Solomos, J. 2007. Immigration, social cohesion and social capital, a critical review. *Critical Social Policy*, 27, 24–49.

Clark, W. 2004. Race, class, and segregation patterns in US immigrant gateway cities. *Urban Affairs Review*, 39(6), 667–88.

Cohen, J.L. and Arato, A. 1999. *Civil Society and Political Theory*. Cambridge, MA: MIT Press.

Conti, C. and Sgritta G.B. 2004. Immigrazione e Politiche Socio-sanitarie, la Salute degli Altri. *Salute e società*, 2.

Conti, C. and Sgritta G.B. (eds) 2004. *Salute e Società. Immigrazione e politiche sociosanitarie. La salute degli altri*. Anno. III (2). Milano: Franco Angeli.

Devadason, R. 2007. *Cosmopolitanism in a Global City, Inclusive Ideals, Exclusive Realities?* Paper presented at the ECPR conference, Pisa, 6–8 September.

Dent, M. 2005. Post-New Public Management in public sector hospitals? The UK, Germany and Italy. *Policy and Politics*, 334, 623–36.

Doern, G.B. and Wilks, S. 1999. *Changing Regulatory Regimes in Britain and North America*. Toronto: University of Toronto Press.

Dunn, J.R. and Dyck, I. 2000. Social determinants of health in Canada's immigrant population, results from the National Population Health Survey. *Social Science & Medicine*, 51(11), 1573–93.

Eade, J. 1997. *Living the Global City: Globalization as Local Process*. London/New York: Routledge.

Eder, K., Giesen, B., Schmidtke, O. and Tambini, D. 2002. *Collective Identities in Action. A Sociological Approach*. London: Ashgate.

Edgington, D., Hanna, B., Hutton, T. and Thompson, S. 2001, *Urban Governance, Multiculturalism and Citizenship in Sydney and Vancouver*. Vancouver Centre of Excellence, RIIM Working Paper Series No. 01–05.

Edwards, C. 2008. Participative urban renewal? Disability, community, and partnership in New Labour's urban policy. *Environment and Planning*, 407, 1664–80.

Ellis, M. and Almgren, G. 2009. Local contexts of immigrant and second-generation integration in the United States. *Journal of Ethnic and Migration Studies*, 35(7), 1059–76.

Elwert, G. 1982. Gesellschaftliche Integration durch Binnenintegration? *Kölner Zeitschrift für Soziologie und Sozialpsychologie*, 4, 717–31.

Enquete-Kommission. 2002. *Zukunft des bürgerschaftlichen Engagements des Deutschen Bundestags. Bericht. Bürgerschaftliches Engagement, auf dem Weg in eine zukunftsfähige Bürgergesellschaft*. Schriftenreihe Band 4 Opladen: Leske und Budrich.

Entzinger, H. 2003. The rise and fall of Multiculturalism: The case of the Netherlands, in *Toward Assimilation and Citizenship, Immigrants in Liberal Nation-States*, edited by C. Joppke and E. Morawska. Basingstoke: Palgrave, 59–86.

Entzinger, H. and Biezeveld, R. 2003. *Benchmarking in Immigrant Integration*. Rotterdam: European Research Centre on Migration and Ethnic Relations.

Esping-Andersen, G. 1990. *The Three Worlds of Welfare Capitalism*. Princeton: Princeton University Press.

Esping-Andersen, G. 2002. A new gender contract, in *Why We Need a New Welfare State*, edited by G. Esping-Andersen, A. Hemerijck, A. and J. Myles. Oxford: Oxford University Press, 68–90.

Esser, H. 2004. Does the "new" immigration require a "new" theory of intergenerational integration? *International Migration Revue*, 38(3), 1126–59.

European Union Minorities and Discrimination Survey. 2009. *Main Results Report*. Vienna: European Union Agency for Fundamental Rights.

Faist, T. and Ozveren, E. (eds) 2004. *Transnational Social Spaces, Agents, Networks and Institutions*. Aldershot: Ashgate.

Falge, C. and Zimmermann, G. 2009. *Interkulturelle Öffnung des Gesundheitssystems*. Frankfurt: Nomos Verlag.

Falge, C., Fischer-Lescano, A. and Sieveking, K. (eds) 2008. *Gesundheit in der Illegalität*. Frankfurt: Nomos.

Favell, A. and Modood, T. 2003. The philosophy of multiculturalism, the theory and practice of normative political theory, in *Contemporary Political Philosophy, a Reader and Guide*, edited by A. Finlayson. Edinburgh: Edinburgh University Press, 484–95.

Favell, A. and Smith, M.P. (eds) 2006. *The Human Face of Global Mobility*. New Brunswick: Transaction Publishers.

Fella, S. and Ruzza, C. 2006. Changing political opportunities and the re-invention of the Italian right. *Journal of Southern Europe and the Balkans*, 8(2) Special Issue, 179–200.

Fella, S. and Ruzza, C. 2007. The National Alliance and Northern League in Italy, Rivals in power, enemies in defeat, in *Identités, Politiques, Sociétés, Espaces, Extrême droite et pouvoir en Europe* [The extreme right parties and power in Europe], edited by P. Poirier and P. Delwit. Bruxelles: Université de Bruxelles, 203–25.

Fennema, M. and Tillie, J. 1999. Political participation and political trust in Amsterdam: Civic Communities and Ethnic Networks. *Journal of Ethnic and Migration Studies*, 25(4), 703–26.

Fennema, M. and Tillie, J. 2001. Civic communities, political participation and political trust of ethnic groups. *Connections*, 24, 26–41.

Fisher, J. 1997. *Nongovernments, NGOs and the Political Development of theThird World*. West Hartford, CT: Kumarian.

Fishkin, J.S. 1993. *Democracy and Deliberation, New Directions for Democratic Reform*. New Haven: Yale University Press.

Foster, L. 1998. *Turnstile Immigration, Multiculturalism, Social Order, and Social Justice in Canada*. Toronto: Thompson Educational Press.

Freeman, G. 1995. Modes of Immigration Politics in Liberal Democratic States. *International Migration Review*, 29, 881–902.

Freeman G. 1998. The decline of sovereignty? Politics and immigration restriction in liberal states, in *Challenge to the Nation State. Immigration in Western Europe and the United States*, edited by C. Joppke. Oxford: Oxford University Press, 86–108.

Freeman, G. 2006. National models, policy types, and the politics of immigration in liberal democracies. *West European Politics*, 29(2), 665–78.

Gagnon, A. 2002. *Responsiveness of the Canadian Health Care System Towards Newcomers*, No. 40, Commission on the Future of Health Care in Canada, Ottawa: Health Canada.

Garbaye R. 2000. Ethnic minorities, cities, and institutions: A comparison of the modes of management of ethnic diversity in a French and a British city, in *Challenging Immigration and Ethnic Relations Politics, Comparative European Perspectives*, edited by R. Koopmans and P. Statham. New York: Oxford University Press, 283–311.

Garbaye, R. 2005. *Getting Into Local Power, the Politics of Ethnic Minorities in British and French Cities*. Boston: Wiley-Blackwell.

Geddes, A. 2003. *The Politics of Migration and Immigration in Europe.* London: Sage.

Geddes, A. 2008. Il rombo dei cannoni? Immigration and the centre-right in Italy. *Journal of European Public Policy*, 153, 349–62.

Geraci S. 1996. *Immigrazione e Salute, un Diritto di Carta? Viaggio nella Normativa Internazionale, Italiana e Regionale*. Rome: Anterem.

Geraci, S. 2005. La Medicina delle Migrazioni in Italia. Un Percorso di Conoscenza e di Diritti. *Studi Emigrazione*, XLII(157), 53–75.

Geraci, S., Bonciani, M. and Martinelli, B. 2010. *La tutela della salute degli immigrati nelle politiche locali*. Rome: Caritas Diocesana di Roma.

Gerber, L. 2004. The visible minority, immigrant, and bilingual composition of ridings and party support in the Canadian federal election of 2004. *Canadian Ethnic Studies*, 381, 65–82.

Giugni, M. and Passy, F. 2004. Migrant mobilization between political institutions and citizenship regimes, a comparison of France and Switzerland. *European Journal of Political Research*, 43, 51–82.

Glaser, B.G. and Strauss, A.L. 1968. *The Discovery of Grounded Theory: Strategies for Qualitative Research*. London: Weidenfeld & Nicolson.

Glick Schiller, N. and Caglar, A. 2009. Towards a comparative theory of locality in migration studies. *Journal of Ethnic and Migration Studies*, 35(2), 177–202.

Glick Schiller, N. and Caglar, A. 2011. *Locating Migration. Rescaling Cities and Migrants.* Ithaca and London: Cornell University Press.

Glick Schiller, N. and Wimmer, A. 2002. Methodological nationalism and beyond: Nation-state building, migration and the social sciences. *Global Networks*, 2, 301–34.

Glick Schiller, N. and Wimmer, A. 2003. Methodological nationalism, the social sciences, and the study of migration, an essay in historical epistemology. *International Migration Review*, 373, 576–610.

Glick Schiller, N., Caglar, A. and Guldbrandsen, T.C. 2006. Beyond the ethnic lens: Locality, globality, and born-again incorporations. *American Ethnologist*, 334, 612–33.

Glick Schiller, N., Nieswand, B., Schlee, G., Darieva, T., Yalçin-Heckmann, L. and Fósztó, L. 2005. Pathways of migrant incorporation in Germany. *Transit*, 1.1, available at: http://escholarship.org/uc/item/90b8w0dh [accessed 10 May 2010].

Goffman, E. 1974. *Frame Analysis*. New York: Harper Row.

Goodman, S. 2007. The politics and policies of immigration in Germany: A rearview look at the makings of a "country of immigration". *German Politics and Society*, 25(4), 99–110.

Green, S. 2004. *The Politics of Exclusion, Institutions and Immigration Policy in Contemporary Germany*. Manchester: Manchester University Press.

Guiraudon, V. 1998. *International Human Rights Norms and their Incorporation, the Protection of Aliens in Europe*. Working Paper. European University Institute, European Forum.

Gunningham, N. 2009. The new collaborative environmental governance: The localization of regulation. *Journal of Law and Society*, 361, 145–66.

Habermas, J. 1996. *Die Einbeziehung des Anderen. Studien zur politischen Theorie*. Frankfurt/M.: Suhrkamp.

Hansen, R. and Koehler, J. 2005. Issue definition, political discourse and the politics of nationality reform in France and Germany. *European Journal of Political Research*, 44(5), 623–44.

Hargreaves, A. and Withol de Wenden, C. 1993. The political participation of ethnic minorities in Europe. *New Community*, 201, 1–18.

Haug, S. 2007. Soziales Kapital als Ressource im Kontext von Migration und Integration, in *Soziale Netzwerke und soziale Ungleichheit. Zur Rolle von Sozialkapital in modernen Gesellschaften*, edited by J. Lüdicke and M. Diewald. Wiesbaden: VS Verlag, 85–111.

Heckmann, F. 1989. Ethnische Kolonien, Schonraum für Integration oder Verstärker der Ausgrenzung? in *Ghettos oder ethnische Kolonien? Entwicklungschancen von Stadtteilen mit hohem Zuwandereranteil*, edited by Forschungsinstitut der Friedrich-Ebert-Stiftung, Abt. Arbeit und Sozialpolitik, Bonn: Friedrich Ebert Stiftung, 29–42.

Heckmann, F. and Schnapper, D. (eds) 2003. *The Integration of Immigrants in European Societies. National Differences and Trends of Convergence*. Stuttgart: Lucius & Lucius.

Hiebert, D. 2005. Migration and the demographic transformation of Canadian cities: The social geography of Canada's major metropolitan centres in 2017, available at: www.canadianheritage.gc.ca/progs/multi/canada2017/5_e.cfm [accessed 23 September 2009].

Hiebert, D. and Sherrell, K. 2009. *The Integration and Inclusion of Newcomers in British Columbia*. Working Paper No. 2009–11, Vancouver, BC, Metropolis British Columbia.

Hollifield, J 1994. *Immigrants, Markets, and States, the Political Economy of Postwar Europe*. Cambridge, MA: Harvard University Press.
Hudson, M., Phillips, J., Ray, K. and Barnes, H. 2007. *Social Cohesion in Diverse Communities*. London: Policy Studies Institute.
Ingrosso, M. 2006. *La Promozione del Benessere Sociale*. Milano: Franco Angeli.
Ireland, P. 1994. *The Policy Challenge of Ethnic Diversity, Immigrant Politics in France and Switzerland*. Cambridge, MA: Harvard University Press.
Jackson, J.S. et al. 2001. Contemporary immigration policy orientations among dominant-group members in Western Europe. *The Journal of Social Issues*, 57(3), 431–56.
Jenson, J. 1989. Paradigms and political discourse: Protectitive legislation in France and the United States before 1914. *Canadian Journal of Political Science*, XXI(2), 235–58.
Johnston, H. 1995. A Methodology for frame analysis: From discourse to cognitive schemata, in *Social Movements and Culture*, edited by H. Johnston and B. Klandermans. London: UCL Press.
Joppke C. (ed.) 1998. *Challenge to the Nation State. Immigration in Western Europe and the United States, 177–221*. Oxford: Oxford University Press.
Joppke, C. 1999. *Immigration and the Nation-State: The United States, Germany, and Great Britain*. Oxford: Oxford University Press.
Joppke, C. 2004. The retreat of multiculturalism in the liberal state, theory and policy. *The British Journal of Sociology*, 55(2), 237–57.
Joppke, C. 2007a. Beyond national models: Civic integration policies for immigrants in Western Europe. *West European Politics*, 30(1), 1–22.
Joppke, C. 2007b. Transformation of immigrant integration: Civic Integration and antidiscrimination in the Netherlands, France, and Germany. *World Politics*, 59(2), 243–73.
Jordan, B. and Düvell, F. 2002. *Irregular Migration: The Dilemmas of Transnational Mobility*. Northampton, MA: Cheltenham Glos Elgar.
Karapin, R. 1999. The politics of immigration control in Britain and Germany, subnational politicians and social movements. *Comparative Politics*, 31(4), 423–44.
Kastoryano, R. 2002. *Negotiating Identities. States and Immigrants in France and Germany.* Princeton and Oxford: Princeton University Press.
Kastoryano, R. 2006. French secularism and Islam, France's headscarf affair, in *Multiculturalism, Muslims and Citizenship*, edited by T. Modood, A. Triandafyllidou and R. Zapata-Barrero. London/New York: Routledge, 57–69.
King, C. and Cruickshank, M. 2010. Building capacity to engage, Community engagement or government engagement? *Community Development Journal*. Advance copy. Available at: http://cdj.oxfordjournals.org/content/early/2010/04/13/cdj.bsq018 [accessed 18 May 2010].
Koopmans, R. 2004. Migrant mobilisation and political opportunities: Variation among German cities and a comparison with the United Kingdom and the Netherlands. *Journal of Ethnic and Migration Studies*, 30(3), 449–70.

Koopmans, R. and Statham, P. 1999. Challenging the liberal nation-state? Postnationalism, multiculturalism, and the collective claims making of migrants and ethnic minorities in Britain and Germany. *American Journal of Sociology*, 105(3), 652–96.

Koopmans, R., Berger, M. and Golonska, C. 2002. *Not a Zero-Sum Game: Ethnic Communities and Political Integration of Migrants in Berlin*. Paper presented at the ECPR Joint Session Turin, Italy, 22–27 March 2002.

Koopmans, R., Statham, P., Giugni, M. and Passy, F. 2005. *Contested Citizenship. Immigration and Cultural Diversity in Europe.* Minneapolis: University of Minnesota Press.

Kosic, A. and Triandafyllidou, A. 2005. *Active Civic Participation of Immigrants in Italy*. Country Report prepared for the European research project, Oldenburg: POLITIS.

Kymlicka, W. 1995. *Multicultural Citizenship*. Oxford: Clarendon.

Kymlicka, W. 1998. *Finding Our Way, Rethinking Ethnocultural Relations in Canada.* Oxford: Oxford University Press.

Kymlicka, W. 2001. *Politics in the Vernacular, Nationalism, Multiculturalism and Citizenship*. Oxford: Oxford University Press.

Laroche, M. 2000. Health status and health services utilization of Canada's immigrant and non-immigrant populations. *Canadian Public Policy*, 261, 51–73.

Levitt, P. 2009. Roots and routes: Understanding the lives of the second generation transnationally. *Journal of Ethnic and Migration Studies*, 35(7), 1225–42.

Levitt, P. and Glick Schiller, N. 2004. Conceptualizing simultaneity, a transnational social field perspective on society. *International Migration Review*, 383, 1002–39.

Ley, D. 2004. Transnational spaces and everyday life. *Transactions of the Institute of British Geographers*, 29(4), 916–33.

Luedtke, A. 2005. The politics of immigration in Western Europe: A Decade of Change. *West European Politics*, 28(3), 680–85.

Lotze, E. 2009. Die Humanitäre Sprechstunde des Gesundheitsamts Bremen – Kommunale Verantwortung für die Gesundheit aller Menschen, in *Gesundheit in der Illegalität. Rechte von Menschen ohne Aufenthaltsstatus*, edited by C. Falge et al. Baden-Baden: NOMOS, 89–95.

Majone, G. 1989. *Evidence, Argument, and Persuasion in the Policy Process*. New Haven, CT: Yale University Press.

Marks, G. 1996. An actor-centred approach to multi-level governance. *Regional and Federal Studies*, 6(2), 20–40.

Marsh, I. 2000. Strategic policy-making and consultation: A second wave in new public management? *Asian Review of Public Administration*, 122, 1–17.

Martiniello, M. 1998. Les Immigrés et les Minorités Ethniques dans les Institutions Politiques, Ethnicisation des Systèmes Politiques Européens ou Renforcement de la Démocratie? *Revue Européenne des Migrations Internationales*, 14(2), 9–17.

Martiniello, M. 2006. Political participation, mobilisation and representation of immigrants and their offspring in Europe, in *Migration and Citizenship, Legal Status, Rights and Political Participation*, edited by R. Bauböck, IMISCOE Reports, Amsterdam: Amsterdam University Press, 83–105.

Martiniello, M. and Statham, P. 1999. Special issue: Ethnic mobilisation and political participation in Europe. *Journal of Ethnic and Migration Studies*, 25(4).

Maturo, A. 2004. Principi e Finalità di Piani di salute, in *Costruire Piani di Salute*, edited by C. Corposanto, L. Fazzi, and A. Scaglia. Milano: Franco Angeli.

Mazey, S. and Richardson, J. 1997. Policy framing: Interest groups and the lead up to the 1996 Inter-Governmental Conference. *West European Politics*, 20(3), 111–33.

McDonald, J.T. and Kennedy, S. 2004 Insights into the "healthy immigrant effect": Health status and health service use of immigrants to Canada. *Social Science and Medicine*, 598, 1613–27.

McLean, C., Campbell, C. and Cornish, F. 2003. African-Caribbean interactions with mental health services in the UK, experiences and expectations of exclusion as reproductive of health inequalities. *Social Science & Medicine*, 563, 657–69.

Mendelberg, T. 2002. The deliberative citizen: Theory and evidence. *Political Decision Making, Deliberation and Participation*, 6, 151–93.

Messina, A.M. 1987. Ethnic minority representation and party competition in Britain, the case of Ealing Borough. *Political Studies*, 35(2), 224–38

Messina, A.M. 1989. *Race and Party Competition in Britain*. Oxford: Oxford University Press.

Messina, A.M. 2006. The political incorporation of immigrants in Europe. Trends and implications, in *The Migration Reader. Exploring Politics and Policies*, edited by A.M. Messina and L. Gallya. London: Lynne Rienner, 470–93.

Messina, A.M. 2007. *The Logics and Politics of Post-WWII Migration to Western Europe*. Cambridge: Cambridge University Press.

Meyer, J.W. and Scott, R.W. (eds) 1983. *Organizational Environments, Ritual and Rationality*. Beverly Hills, CA: Sage.

Milewa, T., Dowswell, G. and Harrison, S. 2002. Partnership, power and the "new" politics of community participation in British health care. *Social Policy and Administration*, 36, 796–809.

Mitchell, K. 2003. *Crossing the Neoliberal Line: Pacific Rim Migration and the Metropolis*. Philadelphia: Temple University Press.

Mitra, D., Jacobsen, M.J., O'Connor, A., Pottie, K. and Tugwell, P. 2006. Assessment of the decision support needs of women from HIV endemic countries regarding voluntary HIV testing in Canada. *Patient Education and Counseling*, 633, 292–300.

Modood, T. et al. 1997. *Ethnic Minorities in Britain*. London: Policy Studies Institute.

Modood, T. 2007. *Multiculturalism: A Civic Idea*. Oxford: Polity Press.

Mohammadzadeh, Z. et al. 2004. *Ältere Migrantinnen und Migranten in Bremen – Lebenssituation, potentielle Versorgungsbedarfe und gesundheitspolitische Perspektiven*. Bremen: Gesundheitsamt.

Morrone A. and Mazzali M. (eds) 2000. *Le Stelle e la Rana. La Salute dei Migranti, Diritti e Ingiustizie*. Milano: Franco Angeli.

Mowbray, M. 2005. Community capacity building or state opportunism? *Community Development Journal*, 403, 255–64.

Newbold K.B. and Danforth J. 2003. Health status and Canada's immigrant population. *Social Science and Medicine*, 57, 1981–95.

O'Toole, T. and Gale, R. 2010. Contemporary grammars of political action among ethnic minority young activists. Special Issue: Migrant Politics and Mobilization, Exclusion, Engagements, Incorporation. *Ethnic and Racial Studies*, 331, 126–43.

Offe, C. 1998. "Homogeneity" and constitutional democracy, coping with identity through group rights. *Journal of Political Philosophy*, 6, 131–41.

Ögelman, N. 2003. Documenting and explaining the persistence of homeland politics among Germany's Turks. *International Migration Review*, 37(1), 163–93.

Okin, S.M. 1999. *Is Multiculturalism Bad for Women?* Princeton: Princeton University Press.

Ossman, S. and Terrio, S. 2006. The French riots, questioning spaces of surveillance and sovereignty. *International Migration*, 44(2), 5–21.

Palidda, R. and Consoli, T. 2006. L'Associazionismo degli Immigrati tra Solidarieta e Integrazione, in *Stranieri in Italia, reti migranti*, edited by F. Decimo and G. Sciortino. Bologna: Il Mulino, 115–49.

Parekh, B. 2000. *Rethinking Multiculturalism. Cultural Diversity and Political Theory*. Cambridge: Polity.

Penninx R. 2004, *Integration: The Role of Communities, Institutions, and the State*. Migration Policy Institute, available at: http://www.migrationinformation.org/Feature/display.cfm?ID=168 [accessed 12 July 2010].

Penninx, R. 2009. *Decentralizing Integration Policies. Managing Migration in Cities, Regions and Localities*. Policy Network Paper, available at: http://www.policy-network.net/publications_download.aspx?ID=3460 [accessed 20 May 2010].

Pero, D. 2005. Left-wing politics, civil society and immigration in Italy: The case of Bologna. *Ethnic and Racial Studies*, 28(5), 832–58.

Pero, D. and Solomos, J. 2010. Introduction: Migrant politics and mobilization; exclusion, engagements, incorporation. *Ethnic and Racial Studies*, 331, 1–18.

Pitkin H.F. 1967. *The Concept of Representation*. Los Angeles, CA: University of California Press.

Poggi, G. 1990. *The State, its Nature, Development and Prospects.* Cambridge: Polity.

Pries, L. 2005. Configurations of geographic and societal spaces: A socio-logical proposal between "methodological nationalism" and the "spaces of flows". *Global Networks*, 5(2), 167–190.

Putnam, R.D. 1995. Bowling alone: America's declining social capital. *Journal of Democracy*, 61, 65–78.

Ray, B. 2003. The role of cities in immigrant integration. *Migration Information Source.* Available at: http://www.migrationinformation.org/feature/display.cfm?ID=167 [accessed 27 July 2007].

Rhodes, R.A.W. (ed.) 2000a. *Transforming British Government. Volume 1: Changing Institutions.* London: Palgrave Macmillan.

Rhodes, R.A.W. (ed.) 2000b. *Transforming British Government. Volume 2: Changing Roles and Relationships*. London: Palgrave Macmillan.

Rogers, A. and Tillie, J. (eds) 2001. *Multicultural Policies and Modes of Citizenship in European Cities*. Aldershot: Ashgate.

Rootes, C. 2007. *Environmental Protest in Western Europe*. Oxford: Oxford University Press.

Rootes, C. 2008. *Acting Locally, Local Environmental Mobilizations and Campaigns*. London: Routledge.

Rosenbaum, A. 2006. Cooperative service delivery, the dynamics of public sector-private sector-civil society collaboration. *International Review of Administrative Sciences*, 72(1), 43–56.

Rummens, J. A. 2003. Identity and Diversity, Overlaps, Intersections and Processes. *Canadian Ethnic Studies*. Special Issue: Intersections of Diversity, 353, 10–25.

Ruzza, C. 2004. *Europe and Civil Society, Movement Coalitions and European Governance*. Manchester: Manchester University Press.

Ruzza, C. 2005. *EU Public Policies and the Participation of Organized Civil Society*. Working Papers del Dipartimento di studi sociali e politici, Milano: Università degli studi di Milano.

Ruzza, C. 2006. Frame analysis, in *Encyclopedia of Language and Linguistics*, edited by K. Brown. Oxford: Elsevier, 3214–21.

Ruzza, C. and Fella, S. 2011. Populism and the Italian right. *Acta Politica*, 1, 1–22.

Ruzza, C. and Schmidtke, O. 1996. The Northern League: Changing friends and foes, and its political opportunity structure, in *Citizenship, Nationality and Migration in Europe*, edited by D. Cesarani and M. Fulbrook. London/New York: Routledge, 179–208.

Saint-Blancat, C. and Friedberg, O. 2005. Why are mosques a problem? Local politics and fear of Islam in northern Italy. *Ethnic and Migration Studies*, 31(6), 1083–1104.

Santoro, W.A. and McGuire, G.M. 1997. Social movement insiders, the impact of institutional activists on affirmative action and comparable worth policies. *Social Problems*, 444, 503–19.

Sassen, S. 1991. *The Global City, New York, London, Tokyo*. Princeton, NJ: Princeton University Press.

Sassen, S. 2000. *Guests and Aliens*. New York: New Press.

Schain, M. 2006. The extreme-right and immigration policy-making: Measuring direct and indirect effects. *West European Politics*, 29(2), 270–89.

Schiffauer, W., Baumann, G., Kastoryano, R. and Vertovec, S. (eds) 2002. *Staat – Schule – Ethnizität. Politische Sozialisation von Immigrantenkindern in vier europäischen Ländern*. Berlin: Waxmann.

Schmidtke, O. 2004. From taboo to strategic tool in politics: Immigrants and immigration policies in German party politics, in *Germany on the Road to Normalcy. Policies and Politics of the Red-Green Federal Government 1998–2002*, edited by W. Reutter, London: Palgrave Macmillan, 161–82.

Schmidtke, O. 2007. (Dis-)Empowering Immigrants in Canada: Political Advocacy of Immigrant and Minority Organisations Promoting Cultural Diversity in the Health Care Sector. *International Journal of Migration, Health and Social Care*, 3(3), 20–28.

Schönwälder, K. 2010. Einwanderer in Räten und Parlamenten. *Aus Politik und Zeitgeschichte*, 46–47, 29–35.

Schönwälder, K. and Kofri, C. 2010. Diversity in Germany's political life? Immigrants in city councils. Max Planck Gesellschaft Working Paper 10–17, Göttingen: MMG.

Schneider, E. et al. 2002. Racial disparities in the quality of health-care for enrollees in Medicare managed care. *Journal of the American Medical Association*, 287, 1288–94.

Schrover M. and Vermeulen F. 2005. Immigrant Organisations. Special Issue of *Journal of Ethnic and Migration Studies*, 31(5).

Siemiatycki, M. and Saloojee, A. 2002. Ethnoracial political representation in Toronto: Patterns and problems. *Journal of International Migration and Integration*, 32, 241–73.

Siemiatycki, M., Rees, T., Ng, R. and Rahi, K. 2003. Integrating community diversity in Toronto, on whose terms? in *The World in a City*, edited by P. Anisef and M. Lanphier. Toronto: University of Toronto Press, 373–456.

Simonet, D. 2008. The New Public Management theory and European health-care reforms. *Canadian Public Administration-Administration Publique Du Canada*, 514, 617–35.

Smith, K.L.W., Matheson, F.I., Moineddin, R. and Glazier, R.H. 2007. Gender, income and immigration differences in depression in Canadian urban centres. *Canadian Journal of Public Health-Revue Canadienne De Sante Publique*, 982, 149–53.

Smith, M.P. 2001. *Transnational Urbanism: Locating Globalization*. Oxford: Blackwell.

Snavely, K. and Desai, D. 2001. Mapping local government-nongovernmental organization interactions: A conceptual framework. *Journal of Public Administration Research and Theory*, 11(2), 245–64.

Sniderman, P. and Hagendoorn, L. 2007. *When Ways of Life Collide, Multiculturalism and its Discontents in the Netherlands*. Princeton: Princeton University Press.

Snow, D.A. 2004. Framing processes, ideology and discursive fields, in *The Blackwell Companion to Social Movements*, edited by D.A. Snow, S.A. Soule and H. Kriesi. Malden, MA and Oxford, UK: Blackwell Publishing, 380–412.

Snow, D.A. and Benford, R.D. 1992. Master frames and cycles of protest, in *Frontiers in Social Movement Theory*, edited by A.D. Morris and C.M. Clurgh Mueller. New Haven, CT: Yale University Press, 133–55.

Soysal, Y.N. 1994. *Limits of Citizenship, Migrants and Postnational Membership in Europe*. Chicago: University of Chicago Press.

Spallek, J. and Razum, O. 2006: Migrantensensible Studiendesigns in der Epidemiologie – Das deutsche Konzept "Staatsangehörigkeit", in *Migrantensensible Studiendesigns zur Repräsentation des Migrationsstatus in der Gesundheitsforschung*. Robert Koch-Institut: Berlin, 23–9.

Stasiulis, D. and Bakan, A. 2003. *Negotiating Citizenship, Migrant Women in Canada and the Global System*. London: Palgrave.

Statham, P., Koopmans, R., Giugni, M. and Passy, F. 2005. Resilient or adaptable Islam? Multiculturalism, religion and migrants' claims-making for group demands in Britain, the Netherlands and France. *Ethnicities*, 5(4), 427–59.

Sundquist, J.A.N. 2001. Migration, equality and access to health care services. *British Medical Journal*, 55, 691–92.

Taylor, M. 2002. Is partnership possible? Searching for a new institutional settlement, in *Urban Governance, Institutional Capacity and Social Milieux*, edited by G. Cars, P. Healey, A. Madanipour, and C. De Magalhaes, Aldershot: Ashgate, 106–24.

Testa, T. 2007. *Professione Volontario*. Roma: Repubblica TV.

Thouez, C. and Channac, F. 2006. Shaping international migration policy: The role of regional consultative processes. *West European Politics*, 29(2), 370–87.

Tiesdell, S. and Allmendinger, P. 2001. Neighbourhood regeneration and New Labour's third way. *Environment & Planning C, Government & Policy*, 19, 903–26.

Tolley, E. 2003. Expressing citizenship through participation, values and responsibilities. *Canadian Diversity*, 2(1), 13–16.

Urbinati, N. 2006. *Representative Democracy, Principles and Genealogy*: Chicago: University of Chicago Press.

Vasta, E. 2007. *Accommodating Diversity: Why Current Critiques of Multiculturalism Miss the Point*. COMPAS Working Paper Series 39. Oxford, COMPAS: University of Oxford.

Vertovec, S. 1998. Multicultural policies and modes of citizenship in European cities. *International Social Science Journal*, 50(2), 187–99.

Vertovec, S. and Wessendorf, S. 2009. *The Multiculturalism Backlash. European Discourses, Policies and Practices*. London/New York: Routledge.

Waldinger, R. 1996. Ethnicity and opportunity in the plural city, in *Ethnic Los Angeles*, edited by R. Waldinger and M. Bozorgmehr. New York: Russell Sage Foundation, 445–70.

Wallace, C. and Pichler, F. 2007. Patterns of formal and informal social capital in Europe. *European Sociological Review*, 23(4), 423–36.

Walker, J. 1991. *Mobilizing Interest Groups in America, Patrons, Professions and Social Movements*. Ann Arbor, MI: University of Michigan Press.

Warren, M. 2001. *Democracy and Association*. Princeton: Princeton University Press.

Werbner, P. 2002. *The Migration Process: Capital Gifts, and Offerings among Overseas Pakistanis*. Oxford: Berg.

Wesselmann, E. and Lindemeyer, T. et al. 2004. *Wenn wir uns nicht verstehen, verstehen wir nichts. Übersetzen im Krankenhaus. Der klinikinterne Dolmetscherdienst*. Frankfurt: Mabusc-Vcrlag.

Wittig, U. et al. 2004. Complaints and health-care system utilisation of ethnic German migrants from the former Soviet Union to Germany and their families. *Gesundheitswesen*, 662, 85–92.

Wimmer, A. 2008. The making and unmaking of ethnic boundaries: A multilevel process theory. *American Journal of Sociology*, 113(4), 970–1022.

Zincone. G. 2001. *Secondo rapporto sull'integrazione degli immigrati in Italia*. Bologna: Il Mulino.

Zincone, G. 2006. The making of policies: Immigration and immigrants in Italy. *Journal of Ethnic and Migration Studies*, 32(3), 347–75.

Policy Documents

ACCÉSSS (2006). RAPPORT ANNUEL. 2005–2006. Montreal: ACCÉSSS.

ACCÉSSS (2007). RAPPORT ANNUEL. 2006–2007. Montreal: ACCÉSSS.

AMSSA (2004). Achieving Equal Access in Health Care. Vancouver: AMSSA.

British Columbia (1996a). Multiculturalism Act [RSBC 1996] CHAPTER 321. Victoria: Queen's Press.

British Columbia (1996b). Human Rights Code [RSBC 1996] CHAPTER 210. Victoria: Queen's Press.

British Columbia (2005). Performance Agreement between the Ministry of Health Services and the Vancouver Coastal Health Authority, April 1, 2005 – March 31, 2006. Victoria, Ministry of Health Services.

Caritas Italiana—Fondazione Migrantes (2010). Rapporto XIX—Immigrazione—Dossier Statistico 2010. Rome.

Council of Europe (1992). Convention on the Participation of Foreigners in Public Life, 5.II.1992, ETS 144, Strasbourg: Council of Europe.

Council of Europe (1999). Political and Social Participation of Immigrants Through Consultative Bodies. CDMG (99) 21. Strasbourg, Council of Europe.

Government of Canada (1982). Charter of Rights and Freedoms, PART I OF THE CONSTITUTION ACT. Ottawa: Government of Canada.

Government of Canada (1988) Multiculturalism Act, R.S., 1985, c. 24 (4th Supp.). Ottawa: Government of Canada.

Quebec (1975). Charter of Human Rights and Freedoms. R.S.Q., chapter C-12.

Quebec (2009) Bill 83: An Act to amend the Act respecting health services and social services and other legislative provisions. Section 433.1

Quebec (2010). An Act respecting health services and social services (2010 update). Available at: http://www2.publicationsduquebec.gouv.qc.ca [accessed 4 January 2011].

Sante Montreal (2004) Interregional Bank of Interpreters, 2003–2004.

Vancouver Coastal Health (2005). Terms of Reference for the VCH Community Advisory Committees. Vancouver: Community Engagement Department.

Vancouver Coastal Health (n.d.). Bridge Community Health Clinic: Primary Health Care for Newcomers to Canada. Vancouver: VCH.

Vicentini, A. and T. Fava (2001). *Le Associazioni di Cittadini Stranieri in Italia.* Venice: Fondazione Corazzin.

Index

Bold page numbers indicate tables.

access to health care *see also* barriers to access
  Canada 155
  equal access as justifying multiculturalism 32
ACCÉSSS (*Alliance des Communautés culturelles pour l'égalité dans la santé et les services sociaux*) 151
advocacy, political
  bottom-up 42
  Canada 52–3, 73–5
  cross-sectoral coalitions 181–2
  degree of involvement by country 63–7, **64**
  Germany 83–5
  health policies, analysis of 43
  Italy 95–100
  key variables 179–84
  as less welcome 103
  location of efforts 102
  low participation of migrants 41
  resonance with health care system imperatives 182–4
  as role of civil society 70
Affiliation of Multicultural Societies and Service Agencies (AMSSA) 77–8
agents of change 171–2
appropriateness of care 32–5
assimilation, return of as discredited 1–2
associations, migrants'
  Canada, role of in 152–3
  cross-sectoral coalitions 181–2
  funding of 57
  Germany 53–9
  Italy 60–1, 95–100, 167–70
  location of advocacy efforts 102
  negative reaction to mobilization 54
  number of 55–6
  orientation towards original country 56, **56**
  representation of 102–03
  as safeguard against state 65
  standards for assessing role of 70–71
  strength and organization of 180–81
  studies of 54
AWO (Workers Welfare Organization) 141–2

barriers to access
  Canada 106, 109, 110–11
  as constantly changing 136–7
  economic issues 107, 113, 132–4
  for female migrants 123
  Germany 106–07, 110
  group-specific differences 114–18
  as important indicators 105
  internal territorial differences 114
  Italy 107, 110, 111–12
  knowledge of services, lack of 106–09
  lack of data on diversity 134–6
  language 117, 118–27, 145
  legal status of immigrants 127–32
  location of services 112–14
  mental health services 110–11
  political factors 114
  preventative programs, lack of use of 109–12
  reasons for 137
  signs in hospitals 123–4
  as similar in different systems 105
  similarity of original country's system 116–17
Baumann, Gerd 20, 20n3
birthing project, community, in Canada 156–7
Blair government *see* New Labour

Bremen Bureau of Public Health (BoH) 140–41
Bridge Clinic, Vancouver 156

Caglar, A. 13n10
Canada
access to services, improving 155
ACCÉSSS (*Alliance des Communautés culturelles pour l'égalité dans la santé et les services sociaux*) 151
advocacy, political 75–8
Affiliation of Multicultural Societies and Service Agencies (AMSSA) 77–8
agents of change 171–2
appropriateness of care 32–5
associations, migrant, role of 152–3
associations as safeguard against state 65
barriers to access 106, 109, 110–11, 112
birthing project, community 156–7
Bridge Clinic, Vancouver 156
change strategies 172–6
Charter of Rights and Freedoms 24n7, 51
civil society
actors 151–3
compared to Italy and Germany 101–02
functions and limits of in 71–3
as kept to a minimum 73
networks and advocacy groups 52–3
representation of migrants 103
community engagement, effectiveness of in 75–8
community groups 151
community health centers 155–6
costs of interpretation services 127
cultural mediation 122–3
degree of involvement 64, **64**
economic issues 132
equal access as justifying multiculturalism 32
group-specific differences 114–15, 115–16
health promotion partnerships 152
Healthiest Babies Possible (HBP) 157
information partnerships 151–2
intercultural approach 26n11
International Bank of Interpreters (IBI) 121–2
interpretation services 36–7, 125, 157–8
intervention groups 159
lack of data on diversity as barrier 134
language 36–7, 121–3
language as barrier to access 125, 126
legal-regulatory framework 148–51
legal status of immigrants 127, 128–9
liaison workers project 154–5
mental health services 110–11, 153
migrant-specific services 153–60
migrants as having responsibility for integration 28–9
Montreal Children's Hospital (MCH) 155
Multicultural Health Fair 77
multiculturalism as dependent on universalism 38
participation by migrants 50–53
practitioners/liaison workers comparison 160
prenatal care 156
settlement services in 9
settlement workers 153–4
signs in hospitals 124
social movement sector 52–3
training, intercultural 158–60
translation services 121–3
understanding of multiculturalism 24–5
Caponio, T. 169
change strategies 172–6
cities
focus on in research 12–13
global 13n10, 14, 14n12
participation of migrants 55
citizens as clients 9, 46
citizenship tests 2
civic multiculturalism 4–5
civil society
advocacy efforts 70, 103
benefits of 48, 101
Canada
actors in 151–3

compared to Italy and Germany 101–02
functions and limits of in 71–3
networks and advocacy groups 52–3
cross-sectoral coalitions 181–2
different conceptualizations of 45
different formations of 49
economic trends, impact of 103
Germany
actors in 141–3
advocacy, political 83–5
Bremer Modell 79
compared to Italy and Canada 101–02
federal/regional/city variations 78–80
functions and limits of 80–83
group formation and engagement 80–83
lack of formalized relationships 85
lack of state involvement 79–80
national model, lack of 85
non-state professional medical associations 78–9
group formation and engagement 80–83
impact of on health policies 44–5
information provision as role 47–8, 70
Italy 60–63
actors 167–70
advocacy, political 95–100
bureaucratic approach of officials 88–9
center-right government, 2008 90–91
compared to Germany and Canada 101–02
consultative forum 88
cooperation with government 86–8
cultural mediation 100–01
functions and limits of in 91–4
Gruppi Regionali Immigrazione e Salute (*GRIS*) 90, 164–5
Gruppo di Lavoro Salute e Immigrazione 88
legislative uncertainty 91
normalization/polarization 91
organization of in 66
and public institutions on policy 165
reduction in participation opportunities 89–90
representation of migrants 92–4
service providers, interaction with 100–01
Società Italiana di Medicina Delle Migrazioni (*SIMM*) 86, 90
New Public Management (NPM) 46
policy learning, fostering of by 47
in policy-making and public administration 45–9
service delivery
centrality of 103
as role 70
states and non-state actors 46
strength and organization of 180–81
structure of 65–6
variables concerning participation 101–02
communal diversity 19n1
communication as challenge to adequate services 35–7
communities, migrant, strength and organization of 179–80
community engagement *see also* civil society
Canada
effectiveness of in 75–8
functions and limits of in 71–3
variation in scope and form 73–5
decentralization of settlement services 9–10
intersection with policy process 8
key elements of strategies 10–11
limitations of research into 5
New Labour's approach 46n3
New Public Management approach 9
trends in 9
urban-centered perspective 5–6
community groups in Canada 151
community health centers in Canada 155–6
cross-sectoral coalitions 181–2
Cruickshank, M. 11
cultural mediation 100–01, 122–3, 166, 171–2

Dachverband Ausländischer Vereine (DAB) 57
data on diversity, lack of as barrier 134–6
decentralization
of government 14
settlement services 9–10
DEVA 80–81, 142
discrimination in Italy 117
diversity, multi-dimensional understanding of 19n1

economic issues as barriers to access 107, 113, 132–4
education
and different groups 116
lack of among immigrants 106–07
emergency services, preferred use of by immigrants 109–12
equal access to health care services 3–4, 30–2 *see also* barriers to access
equality and multiculturalism 19–20
ethnicity, conceptualization of 14
European Union 48

female migrants, barriers to access for 123
frame analysis methodology 15–16

Geraci, S. 113
Germany
advocacy, political 83–5, 102, 181
agents of change 171–2
associations, migrant 53–9
AWO (Workers Welfare Organization) 141–2
barriers to access 110
knowledge of services, lack of 106–07
location of services 112
Bremen Bureau of Public Health (BoH) 140–41
change strategies 172–6
civil society
actors in 141–3
Bremer modell 79
compared to Canada and Italy 101–02
federal/regional/city variations 78–80
functions and limits of 80–83
group formation and engagement 80–83
lack of formalized relationships 85
lack of state involvement 79–80
Migration and Public Health working group 78
national model, lack of 85
non-state professional medical associations 78–9
representation of migrants 103
Council for Integration 57
Dachverband Ausländischer Vereine (DAB) 57
degree of involvement 64, **64**
diversity training 118–19
economic issues 133–4
equal access as justifying multiculturalism 30–31
group-specific differences 115, 116–17
Home Instruction for Parents of Preschool Children (HIPPY) 142
Institut für Psychosoziale Arbeit und Prävention (IPAP) (DEVA) 80–81, 142
insurance, health 141
Interkulturelles Gesundheitnetzwerk Bremen 82
Komijin 143
lack of data on diversity as barrier 134–6
language as barrier to access 118–21, 124–5, 126
language services, lack of in 112
Leben und Arebeiten in Viefalt: Gesundheit Interkulturelle 81–2
legal-regulatory framework 140–41
legal status of immigrants 127–8, 129
mental health services 110, 143
migrant-friendly services 146–8
participation by migrants 53–9
perception of migrants, changes in 84
practitioners and professionals 143–8
psychological counseling in Russian and Turkish 81
Refugio 142–3
rejection of institutional support 57–8
Saglikli Yasa 80

signs in hospitals 124
translation services 35, 118, 119–20
understanding of multiculturalism 25–6, 27–8, 27–9
universalistic values 37–8
Glick Schiller, N. 13–14, 13n10, 22
global cities 13n10, 14, 14n12
government, decentralization of 14
Gruppi Regionali Immigrazione e Salute (GRIS), Italy 90, 164–5
Gruppo di Lavoro Salute e Immigrazione, Italy 88

health
defined as policy sector 69–70
right to 69n1
health care systems
as critical test case 3
equal access 3–4
health promotion partnerships 152
Healthiest Babies Possible (HBP), Canada 157
Heckmann, Friedrich 54
Home Instruction for Parents of Preschool Children (HIPPY) 142

identity, group, as in continuous flux 21
immigrant community, use of term 19n2
inclusion
lack of empirical research 3
use of term in book 2n4
information
Canadian civil society 72–3
lack of data on diversity as barrier 134–6
partnerships in Canada 151–2
provision of as role of civil society 47–8, 70
Institut für Psychosoziale Arbeit und Prävention (IPAP), (DEVA), Germany 80–81, 142
institutional actors 171–2
insurance, health 141
integration of migrants
as challenge for Western societies 1
migrants as having responsibility for (in Canada) 28–9
national background of migrants 116
political, factors impacting 42–3
interculturalism, goal of 26, 26n11
interest groups *see* civil society
Interkulturelles Gesundheitnetzwerk Bremen, Germany 82
International Bank of Interpreters (IBI), Canada 121–2
interpretation services
Canada 36–7, 121–3, 157–8
as challenge 35–7
costs of 126–7
Germany 118, 119–20
lack of in Canada 125
intervention groups 159
interviews 14–15, **15**
Islamic menus 166
Italian Society for Migrants' Medicine 86, 90
Italy
administrative culture 170
advocacy, political 102, 181
agents of change 171–2
associations, migrant, 60–61
barriers to access 110, 111–12
knowledge of services, lack of 107
location of services 112–14
change strategies 172–6
citizenship and immigrations laws 60–61
civil society 60–63
actors 167–70
advocacy, political 95–100
bureaucratic approach of officials 88–9
center-right government, 2008 90–91
compared to Canada and Germany 101–02
consultative forum 88
cooperation with government 86–8
cultural mediation 100–01
development of in 86–91
functions and limits of in 91–4
Gruppi Regionali Immigrazione e Salute (GRIS) 90, 164–5
Gruppo di Lavoro Salute e Immigrazione 88
legislative uncertainty 91

normalization/polarization 91
organization of in 66
and public institutions on policy 165
reduction in participation opportunities 89–90
representation of migrants 92–4, 103
service providers, interaction with 100–01
Società Italiana di Medicina Delle Migrazioni (*SIMM*) 86, 90
costs of interpretation services 127
cultural mediation 166
degree of involvement 64, **64**
economic issues 113, 132–3
equal access as justifying multiculturalism 30
group-specific differences 117
health care as not crucial for migrants 93
health citizenship 87
lack of data on diversity as barrier 136
language 123–4
legal-regulatory framework 160–64
legal status of immigrants 129–31
migrant-specific services 164–7
participation by migrants 60–63
patience of front-line workers, lack of 123
professionals in health care systems 164–5
racism and discrimination 117
signs in hospitals 123
understanding of multiculturalism 25–7, 25n8
universalistic nature of services 165
universalistic values 37–8

Joppke, Christian 2, 6n6, 27n12

King, C. 11
knowledge of services, lack of 106–09
Komijin 143
Koopmans, R. 54–5
Kymlicka, Will 20, 21

language
acquisition of as key in universalism 28
as barrier to access 118–27
Canada 36–7, 121–3
as challenge to adequate services 35–7
costs of interpretation services 126–7
cultural/linguistic translation services 120–21
dependence on family members 125–6
Germany 118–21
Italy 123–4
lack of services in Germany 112
perceptions of as barriers 145
signs in hospitals 123–4
Leben und Arbeiten in Viefalt: Gesundheit Interkulturelle, Germany 81–2
legal-regulatory frameworks
Canada 148–51
Germany 140–41
Italy 160–4
legal status of immigrants 127–32
liaison workers project in Canada 154–5
literacy, lack of among immigrants 106–07
Living and Working in Diversity: Health Intercultural, Germany 81–2
local level, focus on in research 11–14
location of services 112–14

Martiniello, M. 42
mental health services 110–11, 143, 153
methodological nationalism 13–14, 22
methodology 14–16, **15**
migrant-specific services
Canada 153–60
Germany 146–8
Italy 164–7
Modood, Tariq 4–5
Montreal Children's Hospital (MCH) 155
Multicultural Health Fair, Canada 77
multiculturalism
civic 4–5
controversy over 1
and day-to-day practice 21
as dependent on universalism 38
equal access to health care as justifying 30–32
and equality 19–20
as ignoring individual difference 27–8
lack of agency of migrants/minorities 6
migrant health experts, justification of by 31

nationally-specific understandings of 24–9
opposition with universalism 19–21
problems with reforms 22–3
state involvement in Canada 50–53
turn away from 64–5
and universalism, conceptual ambivalence 38
use of term 20n4

National Action Committee on the Status of Women (NAC), Canada 52–3
national models, going beyond 11–14
New Labour 9–10, 10n9, 46n3
New Public Management (NPM) 9, 46

Parekh, B. 55
participation by migrants
Canada 50–53
Germany 53–9
Italy 60–63
perspective diversity 19n1
policy, health
citizens' involvement in, need for 70
civil society
impact of 44–5
opportunities for 45–9
degree of involvement by country 63–7, **64**
as suitable for analysis 43
policy learning 47
political practice by migrants/minorities
civic multiculturalism 4–5
intersection with policy process **8**
limitations of research into 5
urban-centered perspective 5–6
politics
changing opportunity structure 177–9
decentralization of 14
integration, factors impacting 42–3
low participation of migrants 41
prenatal care in Canada 156
pressure groups *see* civil society
preventative programs, lack of use of 109–12
professionals in health care systems 52–3, 171–2
Germany 143–8
Italy 164–5

racism in Italy 117
Refugio 142–3
regulatory frameworks *see* legal-regulatory frameworks
representation of migrants 92–4, 102–03

Saglikli Yasa, Germany 80
Schönwälder, K. 54
service delivery
centrality of 103
as role of civil society 70
service providers, interaction with in Italy 100–01
settlement services, decentralization of 9–10
settlement workers in Canada 153–4
signs in hospitals 123–4
social capital of migrants 107–09
social movement sector in Canada 52–3
social workers 144
Società Italiana di Medicina Delle Migrazioni (*SIMM*), Italy 86, 90
staff, migrant, employment of 144–6
states
associations as safeguard against 65
and multiculturalism 50–53
and non-state actors 46
strategies for change 172–6
sub-cultural diversity 19n1
sub-national governance, importance of 13

training
diversity, in Germany 118–19
intercultural, in Canada 158–60
translation services
Canada 36–7, 121–3, 157–8
as challenge 35–7
costs of 126–7
cultural/linguistic 120–21
Germany 35, 118, 119–20

Universal Declaration of Human Rights 69n1
universalism
access to health care services 3–4
and day-to-day practice 21
as dependent on multiculturalism 38
language acquisition as key 28

and multiculturalism, conceptual ambivalence 38
multiculturalism seen as ignoring individual difference 27–8
opposition with multiculturalism 19–21
urban context 12

Vasta, E. 55

Wimmer, A. 13, 22
women's movement in Canada 52–3
Working Group on Labour, Health and Immigration, Italy 88